The
Complete
Guide to
OPPE

Strategies for Medical Staff Professionals,
Physician Leaders, and Quality Directors

Evalynn Buczkowski, RN, BSN, MS
Valerie Handunge, MA
Wendy R. Crimp, BSN, MBA, CPHQ

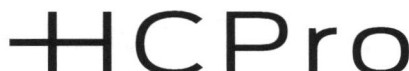

The Complete Guide to OPPE: Strategies for Medical Staff Professionals, Physician Leaders, and Quality Directors is published by HCPro, Inc.

Copyright © 2011 HCPro, Inc.

Cover Image © Kallistova Nina. Used under license from shutterstock.com.

All rights reserved. Printed in the United States of America.   5   4   3   2   1

Download the additional materials of this book at www.hcpro.com/downloads/9567.

ISBN: 978-1-60146-864-2

No part of this publication may be reproduced, in any form or by any means, without prior written consent of HCPro, Inc., or the Copyright Clearance Center (978/750-8400). Please notify us immediately if you have received an unauthorized copy.

HCPro, Inc., provides information resources for the healthcare industry. HCPro, Inc., is not affiliated in any way with The Joint Commission, which owns the JCAHO and Joint Commission trademarks.

Evalynn Buczkowski, RN, BSN, MS, Author

Valerie Handunge, MA, Author

Wendy R. Crimp, BSN, MBA, CPHQ, Contributing Author

Elizabeth Jones, Associate Editor

Julie A. McCoy, Managing Editor

Erin E. Callahan, Associate Editorial Director

Mike Mirabello, Senior Graphic Artist

Matt Sharpe, Production Manager

Shane Katz, Art Director

Jean St. Pierre, Senior Director of Operations

Advice given is general. Readers should consult professional counsel for specific legal, ethical, or clinical questions. Arrangements can be made for quantity discounts. For more information, contact:

HCPro, Inc.

75 Sylvan Street, Suite A-101

Danvers, MA 01923

Telephone: 800/650-6787 or 781/639-1872

Fax: 800/639-8511

E-mail: *customerservice@hcpro.com*

Visit HCPro online at: *www.hcpro.com* and *www.hcmarketplace.com*

Rev. 03/2012

50792

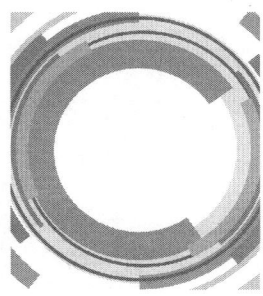

Contents

CONTENTS

© 2011 HCPro, Inc.   THE COMPLETE GUIDE TO OPPE

CONTENTS

CONTENTS

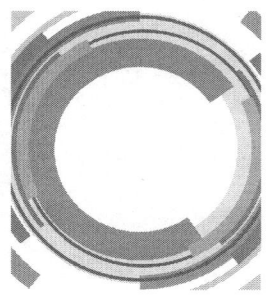

Figure List

FIGURE LIST

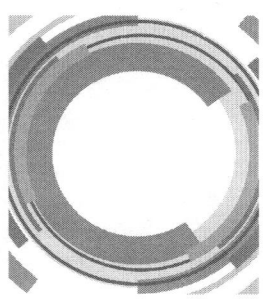

About the Authors

Evalynn Buczkowski, RN, BSN, MS, Author

Evalynn Buczkowski, RN, BSN, MS, is regional director, clinical performance support at Henry Ford Macomb (MI) Hospitals. In this role, she provides leadership for the clinical and operational aspects of clinical quality, clinical informatics, public reporting/pay for performance, accreditation, medical affairs including credentialing and peer review, case management, utilization review, social work, and infection prevention.

She has 25 years of healthcare experience in management, accreditation and regulatory compliance, quality, and performance improvement. Previous to her current position she was responsible for quality and performance improvement operations, clinical integration and nursing professional practice, and nursing education.

Buczkowski received a bachelor of science degree in nursing from Northern Michigan University and a master of science degree in health service administration from the University of Detroit.

She is an active member of the Michigan Health and Hospital Association's Quality and Accountability Committee.

Valerie Handunge, MA, Author

Valerie Handunge, MA, is a senior healthcare strategy and operations consultant with Deloitte Consulting. Her expertise is in accountable care solutions, working with large health systems to address care delivery quality, utilization effectiveness, and physician alignment.

Prior to joining Deloitte Consulting, Handunge was a director with the Advisory Board Company. In this capacity, she provided leadership for business intelligence technology implementations with more than 50 domestic and international hospitals, focusing on physician performance improvement, clinical integration and surgery, and emergency department operational efficiencies. She played an instrumental role in developing the service model for The Advisory Board Company's Crimson ongoing professional practice evaluation module resulting in documented work flow efficiencies and time savings. She has presented at numerous national conferences on OPPE best practices.

She holds a master's degree from the Pennsylvania State University.

Wendy R. Crimp, BSN, MBA, CPHQ, Contributing Author

Wendy R. Crimp, BSN, MBA, CPHQ, is the consulting practice director for The Crimp Resource Group. During her more than 30 years of experience in the healthcare industry, her extensive operational and project management experience has provided an excellent framework for understanding organizational requirements needed to achieve successful management outcomes. She has provided consulting services to hospitals, health systems, municipal public health agencies, medical groups, payers, and universities. Her services have included development and implementation of both operational and clinical quality improvement programs; management of organizations in transition; interim and long-term operations planning; organizational restructure; operations cost management; work flow redesign; and optimizing the use of technology. She is a content expert in the area of clinical quality improvement, credentialing, privileging, and peer review. She has authored numerous articles published in a variety of trade journals, Web resources, and books. She is a regular speaker at national and state conferences.

Crimp received a master's in business administration from the University of California at Irvine and a bachelor of science degree, with distinction, in nursing from California State University of Long Beach. She has an active registered nursing license and is certified in public health in the state of California. She is also a Certified Professional in Healthcare Quality (CPHQ).

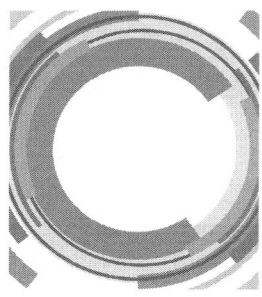

Acknowledgments

This book includes descriptions of the Henry Ford Health System, particularly the Henry Ford Macomb Hospital's work on physician alignment and OPPE-compliant reporting with The Advisory Board Company, a research, consulting, and technology services firm partnering with more than 3,000 of the world's leading healthcare organizations.

In addition to the insights drawn from Henry Ford's OPPE experience, many of the recommendations profiled within are based on research interviews with Advisory Board members who have adopted progressive OPPE processes that provide a meaningful platform for engaging physicians in performance improvement.

The Crimson physician performance technologies support the Henry Ford Macomb Hospital's OPPE reporting for both employed and independent physicians as part of a comprehensive clinical integration initiative. The institution joined the Crimson cohort that has grown to over 500 individual hospitals using business intelligence technology and best practice implementation, dedicated utilization support, and best practice research in care delivery to serve over 130,000 physician users. Author Valerie Handunge played an instrumental role in developing the service model for the Crimson OPPE module, which is utilized by the Henry Ford Health System.

About the Advisory Board Company

The Advisory Board Company is a global research, consulting, and technology firm helping healthcare and university executives to better serve patients and students. The firm provides strategic guidance, actionable insights, Web-based software solutions, and comprehensive implementation and management services. To learn more about The Advisory Board's Crimson services or best practice research programs, visit *www.advisory.com*.

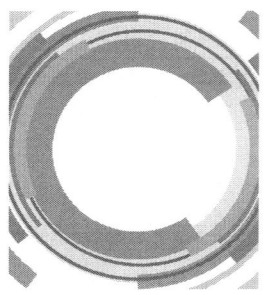

Continuing Education Information

National Association Medical Staff Services (NAMSS)

This program has been approved by the National Association Medical Staff Services for five continuing education units. Accreditation of this educational program in no way implies endorsement or sponsorship by NAMSS.

Continuing Education Instructions

To be eligible to receive your continuing education credits for this activity, you are required to do the following:

1. Read the book, *The Complete Guide to OPPE*.

2. Complete the continuing education exam by visiting the link provided below. You must receive a score of at least 80% to pass.

3. Provide your contact information, including e-mail address, at the end of the exam.

4. Upon successful completion of the exam, you will receive an e-mail with a link to your continuing education certificate. Save this e-mail in case you need to reprint your certificate in the future.

 © 2011 HCPro, Inc.

To start the continuing education exam, copy and paste the following link into your browser:

www.hcpro.com/OPPE/e1

NOTES:

If you cannot access the online continuing education exam, contact customer service at 877/727-1728, and a copy of the exam can be e-mailed to you. Return the exam by mail or fax upon completion.

The Complete Guide to OPPE and associated exam are intended for individual use only. If you want to provide this continuing education exam to other staff members, contact HCPro's customer service department at 877/727-1728. The exam fee schedule is as follows:

Exam Quantity	Fee
1	$0
2–25	$15 per person
26–50	$12 per person
51–100	$8 per person
101+	$5 per person

Learning objectives

Chapter 1

After reading this chapter, you will be able to:

- Discuss The Joint Commission and other regulatory requirements for OPPE

- Explain how OPPE is an extension of healthcare reform and other national quality initiatives

- Identify challenges organizations face when implementing an OPPE process

Chapter 2

After reading this chapter, you will be able to:

- Outline the responsibilities of the OPPE task force

- Compare potential frameworks for the OPPE process

- Define the scope of the OPPE process

- Develop an OPPE policy

Chapter 3

After reading this chapter, you will be able to:

- Construct a communication plan regarding the OPPE implementation

- Determine who needs training on OPPE and what that training should include

- Identify strategies and responses for practitioner pushback

Chapter 4

After reading this chapter, you will be able to:

- Distinguish between rate, rule, and review indicators

- Develop a plan for identifying and evaluating potential indicators

- Create an indicator inventory

- Select indicators based on their validity, feasibility of collection, and relevance

Chapter 5

After reading this chapter, you will be able to:

- Determine when perception should be used

- Distinguish between different types of perception data

- Identify methods for gathering data from perceivers

Chapter 6

After reading this chapter, you will be able to:

- Define relative-action thresholds, fixed-action thresholds, and standard deviation thresholds

- Adjusting data for patient severity/acuity and case complexity

- Identify resources for establishing appropriate thresholds

- Select thresholds based on indicator type

- Use thresholds to interpret variation

Chapter 7

After reading this chapter, you will be able to:

- Discuss why attribution is a challenge in many hospitals

- Identify strategies for solving data integrity issues

- Develop an attribution process at your organization

Chapter 8

After reading this chapter, you will be able to:

- Define why obtaining data for low-volume practitioners and advanced practice professionals is difficult

- Identify data sources and managing low-volume practitioners

- Address low-volume practitioners in the OPPE policy

- Select indicators for APPs with supervised privileges

Chapter 9

After reading this chapter, you will be able to:

- Appraise potential structures for the OPPE reports

- List key elements to include in the OPPE reports

- Select data elements and supporting materials to include in the OPPE reports to facilitate understanding by practitioners

- Conduct a pilot test for the OPPE reports

Chapter 10

After reading this chapter, you will be able to:

- Create a timeline for delivering OPPE reports

- Appraise methods for delivering the OPPE reports

Chapter 11

After reading this chapter, you will be able to:

- Establish a process for reviewing OPPE data

- Differentiate between process deficiencies and practitioner performance issues

- Employ strategies for carrying out performance improvement conversations with practitioners

Chapter 12

After reading this chapter, you will be able to:

- Discuss the process for FPPE at initial privileges

- Identify strategies for carrying out FPPE when performance issues are identified

DOWNLOAD YOUR MATERIALS NOW

Visit the link listed below to download customizable versions of many of the sample forms and tools available in this book.

www.hcpro.com/downloads/9567

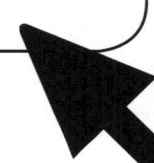

Thank you for purchasing this product!

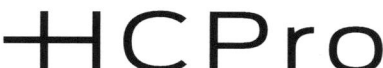

Developing a Strategy for OPPE

CHAPTER

1

The Impetus for Practitioner Performance Improvement

The primary purpose of this book is to support hospital administrative departments and medical staffs as they develop and operationalize an ongoing professional practice evaluation (OPPE) program. Although The Joint Commission introduced OPPE in 2007 (Standard MS.08.01.03), many organizations still struggle to create a meaningful and efficient program given organizational constraints of resources and time, a lack of clear direction, and misconceptions that the program must be created from scratch.

The crux of OPPE is to improve patient care through practitioner performance improvement (PI), which many hospitals already do to some degree through performance feedback reporting at the individual practitioner or aggregate group level, quality/PI projects, and existing credentialing efforts. OPPE requires that these existing initiatives are streamlined and improved into a holistic, systematic, and timely process improvement exercise to be applied at the level of the individual practitioner. This is no easy task.

This book is designed to help organizations through the nuts and bolts of:

- Bringing together the right stakeholders to create an OPPE task force or project team

- Creating a formalized organizational OPPE policy

- Defining clinical, organizational, and departmental goals and metrics

- Selecting meaningful indicators within a competency framework and gathering data for those indicators from various sources

- Proactively analyzing and addressing inherent problems, such as the attribution of data

- Establishing performance thresholds to identify opportunities for PI

- Assessing performance in a structured manner and intervening when practitioners have performance concerns, which may potentially lead to focused professional practice evaluation(s) (FPPE)

- Delivering reports to practitioners and conducting meaningful dialogue around report content and opportunities for improvement

- Communicating a positive message about PI to practitioners

- Determining methods for OPPE for low-volume providers and advanced practice professionals

Before jumping in, it is important to understand the OPPE mandate.

The OPPE Mandate and Requirements

Hospitals appear to be struggling with OPPE for a variety of reasons. Before exploring the challenges, it is important to understand the mandate. The Joint Commission's Standard MS.08.01.03 requires hospitals to monitor the performance of individual practitioners on an ongoing basis, rather than simply every two years when they are due for reappointment. This change in the requirement resulted in:

- Increased frequency of practitioner assessment, which encourages organizations to take steps to improve performance on a more timely basis

- Improved accuracy of credentialing and privileging decisions based on objective competency data

- Expansion of the scope and breadth of practitioner assessment

- Increased practitioner awareness and participation with regard to personal performance analytics

According to The Joint Commission, OPPE information must be factored into the medical staff's decision to allow a practitioner to maintain, revise, or revoke existing privilege(s) prior to or at the time of renewal. Standard MS.08.01.03 requires the following:

- The medical staff must define a process to evaluate each practitioner's professional practice

- Individual departments determine the data collected for evaluation, and the medical staff approves the selected data

- The medical staff use the information gained from OPPE to continue, limit, or revoke existing privileges

It is important to note that the standard does not require hospitals to proactively share evaluations with practitioners; however, if hospitals are to hold practitioners accountable for their quality of care, it is unfair to do so without complete transparency. For simplicity, the temptation is for hospitals to share evaluations only when performance issues are identified; however, this perpetuates the image that OPPE is a punitive process. The authors support organizations in their efforts to share reports with each privileged practitioner.

Practitioner Performance Improvement Goes Beyond OPPE

What is the driving force for PI for hospitals and practitioners beyond simply meeting OPPE requirements? The world of healthcare is changing drastically on many levels. One of the biggest changes is the increased focus by regulatory agencies and the public on quality improvement expectations. Let's take a closer look at the significance of OPPE within the realm of new healthcare regulations, changing payment structures, and healthcare consumer expectations for transparency.

Previously, regulatory and accreditation bodies required medical staffs to evaluate practitioners for renewal of privileges every 24 months. However, the new competency management trend is continuous performance monitoring. For example, at the same time The Joint Commission introduced OPPE, the American Board of Medical Specialties (ABMS) established the annual maintenance of board certification requirements, and the National Practitioner Data Bank (NPDB) initiated the Proactive Data Service, which facilitates real-time monitoring of adverse actions taken against practitioners. It is clear that the industry is driving toward increasingly frequent performance monitoring, which decreases lag time between the reporting of performance information and taking actions to continue, modify, or revoke authorization for clinical practice. For hospital providers, this expectation for continuous monitoring involves conducting OPPE on privileged practitioners. OPPE challenges organizations to evaluate performance and act on information received regarding practitioner performance with greater frequency.

Regulatory requirements from The Joint Commission, CMS, DNV, HFAP, and other regulators

The Joint Commission might have one of the strictest practitioner competency management standards, but other regulators are not far behind. OPPE is a mandate rooted in this new culture of transparency and demands to improve patient care through demonstrated quality and PI. The Centers for Medicare & Medicaid Services (CMS), The Joint Commission, Det Norske Veritas (DNV), and other governing bodies are all pushing for similar results through a variety of mechanisms. Although OPPE is a Joint Commission requirement, other healthcare regulators and accrediting bodies appear to have similar standards that necessitate a process similar to OPPE.

CMS' *Conditions of Participation* (*CoP*) and interpretive guidelines require organizations to develop a clinical competence framework to perform privilege evaluations at a time period not to exceed 24 months. In addition, under sections relating to quality assessment and PI, the *CoP* requires that "the hospital must develop, implement, and maintain an effective, ongoing, hospital-wide, data-driven quality assessment and performance improvement program."

With that said, hospitals accredited by The Joint Commission will not be the only organizations that will benefit from the concepts shared in this book. Hospitals that are accredited by the DNV or the Healthcare Facilities Accreditation Program (HFAP), which are also subject to direct surveys by CMS, will also find the concepts to be of value as they strive to increase the efficiency and effectiveness of their practitioner competency management programs and demonstrate compliance with CMS standards.

Prior to 2007, hospitals responded to both CMS and Joint Commission requirements by implementing a system for reappointment profiling, whereby they evaluated and acted on practice data related to practitioner performance every 24 months at reappointment. In 2007, with the introduction of OPPE, Joint Commission standards became much more prescriptive with regard to both the need for actionable performance data and the requirement to formally evaluate clinical competence more often than every 24 months. Because ongoing monitoring of clinical competence is a higher standard than evaluating clinical competence every 24 months, there has been some speculation about whether this trend might eventually lead to the elimination of the 24-month reappointment.

New payment structures are tied to quality of care

OPPE affects not only patient care, but also hospital and practitioner reimbursement. With healthcare reform, the focus has turned to reimbursement rooted in quality of care as opposed to the fee-for-service models of the past. Pay-for-performance, bundled payments, and shared savings models encourage organizations to reduce variations in quality and utilization and to standardize care around best practices. Organizations that manage costs well while maintaining high quality standards will thrive best under these models.

Based on these payment models, there is an increased likelihood that payer contracts and agreements will be negotiated based on quality data. An early example is the hospital inpatient value-based purchasing program, which CMS proposed in January 2011.

THE IMPETUS FOR PRACTITIONER PERFORMANCE IMPROVEMENT

According to this proposal, the program will be implemented in fiscal year 2013 and will make value-based incentive payments to acute care hospitals based either on how well hospitals perform on certain quality measures or how much their performance improves on certain quality measures. The greater a hospital's performance outcomes or improvement during the performance period beginning July 1, 2011, for a defined period, the higher the hospital's value-based incentive payment for the fiscal year would be.

Many hospital leaders aspire for greater transparency and analysis of individual practitioner performance, believing that this focus would significantly assist hospital quality improvement efforts and promote the understanding of resource consumption, clinical quality, and utilization patterns to improve clinical efficiency. Some hospitals and practitioners are willing to go to greater depths. Hospitals with employed practitioners (especially hospitalists) are incorporating quality and performance goals into their employment contracts, often tied to bonus structures. It only makes sense to include these same metrics in their OPPE programs.

Several larger hospital systems are forming practitioner driven, clinically integrated accountable care organizations (ACO) focused on delivering higher quality care while managing medical costs. These programs measure performance across key competency areas very similar to OPPE. The goal is to negotiate payer contracts based on quality and outcomes of care, and many ACOs are tying bonus payments to practitioners based on performance. Through such initiatives, hospitals and practitioners hope to provide optimal value to patients, payers, and employers through collaborative best practices, evidence-based medicine, and improved efficiencies.

Why Should Practitioners Care About OPPE?

Why should practitioners care about OPPE? Hospitals, payers, and patients are making conscious efforts to align with practitioners based on quality of care, outcomes, and performance. OPPE gives practitioners the framework to proactively manage their data in this era of transparency. Patients have greater access to practitioner quality and performance data. As the consumers of healthcare services, technology-savvy patients are accessing performance data through websites with paid subscriptions, such as *www.ucomparehealthcare.com* and *www.HealthGrades.com*. Responding to the need in the market, other media sources are providing access to healthcare data for free. *USA Today* allows readers to review hospital readmission rates and mortality rankings for common diagnoses, such as pneumonia, congestive heart failure, and acute myocardial infarction.

Insurance companies are also encouraging patients to make educated decisions when choosing practitioners. Many insurers (e.g., United Healthcare, Aetna's Aexcel®) provide practitioner ratings directly on their websites to guide patients to practitioners with better quality outcomes and more efficient cost of care.

CMS already shares data publicly through Hospital Compare (*www.hospitalcompare.hhs.gov*) and is moving toward sharing core measures and more detailed practitioner-level quality data with the public through the Physician Compare (*www.medicare.gov/find-a-doctor*).

To simply frame OPPE as a regulatory compliance mandate is missing the mark of its intent. OPPE is fundamental to a robust practitioner PI framework and a cultural shift toward more data-driven practices. It is imperative that the OPPE model at every organization creates a meaningful quality framework that is aligned with organizational strategy and reporting initiatives, and is directly connected to organizational improvement goals in patient care and clinical outcomes.

Why Do Organizations Struggle With OPPE?

For many organizations, an OPPE program is the first systematic process for broad scale practitioner performance improvement. Organizations run into common pitfalls that often hamper the progress of OPPE, particularly when selecting indicators, reviewing reports, and engaging practitioners. The following are some common mistakes that medical staffs make when implementing OPPE programs.

- **Jumping to tasks (such as selecting indicators) without defining the organizational vision and quality goals for OPPE.** Without a compelling reason for the OPPE program, practitioners may not be receptive to how the program will be implemented. This lack of direction leads to difficulty in selecting meaningful indicators. During the indicator selection process, ask the question, "Does this indicator measure performance that aligns with the organization's or department's vision and goals?"

- **Holding one group accountable for creating the OPPE program.** At some organizations, medical staff leaders coordinate the entire process, whereas at others, the quality and performance improvement departments or the medical staff services department are responsible for data collection and report evaluations. Rather than being a segregated effort, organizations will benefit most if medical staff leaders and the appropriate administrative department work together as they bring different skills and knowledge to the table.

- **Failing to allocate appropriate resources up front.** OPPE requires increased staff resources, and excluding certain stakeholders can be detrimental to the program's success. Not involving medical staff leaders up front may result in a lack of support for the program. Not involving clinical informatics and information technology (IT) resources up front may cause the medical staff to select indicators that are not feasible to collect. Chapter 2 discusses important stakeholders to involve and how to set expectations regarding roles and responsibilities.

- **Selecting indicators and thresholds in a vacuum.** Although it is important for each department to determine the indicators that best evaluate practitioners' performance, working in silos often duplicates efforts and leads to inconsistent indicator definitions and fragmented priorities. Encourage coordination across specialties to allow for collective learning and collaboration. Consider grouping related specialties, such as family practice and internal medicine, so they are selecting indicators together or sharing knowledge between groups.

- **Failing to assign performance thresholds or triggers to indicators.** Failing in this area impedes the ability to apply a fair and equitable performance expectation across a group of practitioners. It also prevents the medical staff from systematically acting on information received via the OPPE process and does not conform to current requirements.

- **Basing indicators on low-integrity data.** Whether the data are untimely, inconsistently captured, gleaned from an insufficient sample size, or simply riddled with data integrity issues, the resulting indicators will not meet accepted standards for validity. During indicator selection and report evaluations, it is crucial to scrutinize the accuracy and reliability of the data.

- **Failing to identify deficiencies in the current program and addressing practitioner skepticism.** Practitioners may be skeptical of the new OPPE program based on their experiences with the previous program for reappointment profiling. For example, they may feel that the data provided was not helpful in determining clinical competence relative to the privileges requested. If an OPPE program is to be credible, it is important to identify deficits in the existing program for reappointment profiling so that the medical staff does not make the same mistakes in the development of the OPPE program.

- **Failing to effectively engage practitioners in OPPE.** Medical staffs often make the mistake of spending a lot of time developing an OPPE process, but they fail to collaborate with practitioners to identify clinically unnecessary variation. Once the process is implemented, they are disappointed with the lack of improved clinical outcomes and view the OPPE process as not worth the time or resources spent.

- **Failing to provide effective communication and education regarding OPPE.** If medical staff members do not understand the intentions of OPPE, they may push back or appear disinterested or uncooperative.

 © 2011 HCPro, Inc.

Building a Successful OPPE Program

As with any project, setting a strong foundation and support structure for your OPPE project is key to success. Fundamental to this initiative are the following tasks:

- Create an OPPE task force

- Develop an OPPE task force or committee charter that identifies the members of the task force, scope of business, authority, and reporting relationship

- Develop a framework for OPPE

- Align existing processes with the new OPPE program, including privileging, credentialing, peer review, core measures, and any product line quality improvement activities that may exist

Creating an OPPE Task Force

Although the structure of every organization varies, developing an OPPE program requires cross-departmental collaboration. The best way to facilitate collaboration is to create an OPPE task force composed of members from several departments.

The purpose of the OPPE task force is to:

- Direct the selection of indicators and thresholds

- Guide the resolutions of data integrity issues and concerns around attribution

- Help design the structure and format of the OPPE reports

- Define the OPPE performance evaluation process

- Define the focused professional practice evaluation (FPPE) process

- Develop the communications plan

- Develop the organization's OPPE policy

- Ensure that the OPPE process reflects the needs and requirements of privilege holders by involving clinical leadership in the entire process

The OPPE task force should be interdisciplinary, meaning that it must contain representatives from the relevant administrative departments at the hospital as well as the medical staff. This includes:

- Administrative physician leaders such as the chief medical officer (CMO), vice president of medical affairs (VPMA), or medical director

THE COMPLETE GUIDE TO OPPE

- Quality department, performance improvement, and medical staff services department representatives (if these departments are separate)

- Chief of staff (particularly if an administrative physician leader role does not exist at your hospital)

- Other key physician executives and medical staff leaders who need to be involved in the OPPE planning process

- Medical informatics/information technology (IT) department representatives

- Medical record coders

It is crucial that medical informatics/IT staff be present during OPPE discussions, particularly as groups select indicators. IT staff will have insight into what data is available electronically within the organization's existing data systems/repositories and will be able to analyze the integrity of the data (particularly by capturing rates for indicators under consideration). IT staff may also be able to set up new infrastructure to capture indicators of interest and provide alternatives when data limitations exist.

Because OPPE is meant to be a practitioner-led initiative, a physician leader should chair the OPPE task force and have administrative support throughout the process. Selecting a physician leader as chair of the task force makes it clear who is responsible and accountable for the development of the OPPE program. Typically, this is the CMO or VPMA (or a medical staff leader if a physician executive role does not exist at your organization).

Once the OPPE task force members have been selected, define the roles and responsibilities of each team member. You may ask additional participants to attend task force meetings or

 © 2011 HCPro, Inc.

to take on projects for topic-specific work. For example, a surgical service administrative leader may assist in developing indicators for procedural practitioners.

TIP

Soon after identifying task force members, schedule recurring task force meetings. This ensures members will have protected time that they can dedicate to building or revamping the OPPE program.

Developing a Framework for OPPE

When The Joint Commission first published the OPPE standards, it provided little guidance for hospitals on how to operationalize the OPPE process. Recently, The Joint Commission, other accrediting bodies, and payers established prescriptive guidelines for conducting OPPE for each privilege holder.

In 2011, The Joint Commission published a *BoosterPak* that provides advice for designing and implementing OPPE and FPPE standards. The Joint Commission references the Accreditation Council for Graduate Medical Education (ACGME) and the American Board of Medical Specialties' (ABMS) general competencies as a potential framework for the type of data collected on practitioners who are credentialed and privileged through the medical staff. The six core competencies are:

- Medical/clinical knowledge

- Practice-based learning and improvement

- Interpersonal and communication skills

- Professionalism

- Systems-based practice

- Patient care

The six competency domains provide a context or framework for identifying and developing indicators. These competencies do not exist in silos—many overlap. As such, indicators may relate to more than one domain. Figure 2.1 provides definitions of each of the six competency areas and examples of indicators for each area.

The OPPE task force may choose another framework to measure competency. The American College of Physician Executives developed a competency framework, which The Greeley Company, a division of HCPro, Inc., the publisher of this book, has adopted. See Figure 2.2 for this competency framework.

FIGURE 2.1

SIX CORE COMPETENCIES AND SAMPLE INDICATORS

	Competency area	Demonstration of competency	Sample indicators
Hospital-level indicators Select the same indicators for all physicians at the hospital. If you are a system and your OPPE program is at the system level (which is recommended), select the same indicators for all physicians at the system.	**Medical/Clinical Knowledge** Demonstrated knowledge of established and evolving biomedical, clinical, and social sciences, and the application of their knowledge to patient care and the education of others	Use evidence-based guidelines when available, as recommended by the appropriate specialty, in selecting the most effective and appropriate approaches to diagnosis and treatment	• Number of continuing medical education (CME) credits earned in established time frame, aligned with privileging criteria or appropriate to area of practice • Results of retrospective case/chart review focused on appropriateness of care • Performance on simulators • Board certification
	Practice-Based Learning and Improvement Use of scientific evidence and methods to investigate, evaluate, and improve patient care	Review individual and specialty/group aggregate data for all general competencies, and use this data for self-improvement to continuously improve patient care	• Dating/timing/signing of all orders • Compliance with established evidence-based practice guidelines • Appropriate drug use—VTE prophylaxis, ASA on admission for AMI patients, statins at discharge for all AMI patients

 © 2011 HCPro, Inc. THE COMPLETE GUIDE TO OPPE

FIGURE 2.1

SIX CORE COMPETENCIES AND SAMPLE INDICATORS (CONT.)

	Competency area	Demonstration of competency	Sample indicators
	Interpersonal and Communication Skills Demonstrated ability to establish and main-tain professional relationships with patients, families, and other members of healthcare teams	Communicate clearly with other physicians and caregivers, patients, and patients' families through appropriate oral and written methods to ensure accurate transfer of information	• Illegible orders • Timeliness of history and physical examinations • Patient satisfaction with physician communication • Incident reports that reflect physician unwillingness to cooperate • Compliments from patients, family, staff
	Professionalism Demonstrated com-mitment to continuous professional develop-ment, ethical practice, sensitivity to diversity, and a responsible attitude toward pa-tients, the profession, and society	• Act in a professional, respectful manner at all times to enhance a spirit of cooperation and mutual respect and trust among members of the patient care team • Respond promptly to requests for patient care needs	• Validated incidents of inappropriate behavior • Responsiveness to emergency depart-ment (ED) call, ED call episodes of noncompliance • Meeting attendance • Medical record suspensions • Number of delin-quency warnings • Number of unsafe/do not use abbreviations

 © 2011 HCPro, Inc.

FIGURE 2.1

SIX CORE COMPETENCIES AND SAMPLE INDICATORS (CONT.)

	Competency area	Demonstration of competency	Sample indicators
		• Respect patients' rights by discussing unanticipated adverse outcomes and by not discussing patient care information and issues in public settings • Participate in emergency room call coverage as determined by medical staff policy	• Percentage of no show/ late/cancellations to scheduled procedures or office visits
Department-specific indicators Select the same indicators for your medicine, surgery, and OB/ GYN departments/ servicelines	**Systems-Based Practice** Demonstrated understanding of patient care systems in which healthcare is provided, and the ability to apply this knowledge to improve and optimize healthcare	• Strive to provide cost-effective quality patient care by cooperating with efforts to manage the use of valuable patient care resources • Participate in the hospital's efforts and policies to maintain a patient safety culture, reduce medical errors, meet National Patient Safety Goals, and improve quality	• Severity-adjusted average length of stay • Pharmacy cost per case • Hand-washing observation data • Number of as needed (PRNs) without indication • Percentage of e-prescribing use • CPOE rates

FIGURE 2.1

SIX CORE COMPETENCIES AND SAMPLE INDICATORS (CONT.)

	Competency area	Demonstration of competency	Sample indicators
Specialty-specific indicators Select indicators relevant to individual specialties and if there are specialties that provide similar care (e.g., internal medicine and family practice) select the same indicators for groups of similar specialties at the same time. Consider working with small groups of specialties at a time.	**Patient Care** Delivery of compassionate, appropriate, and effective patient care that is effective for promoting health, preventing illness, treating disease, and providing comfort at the end of life	• Achieve patient outcomes that meet or exceed generally accepted medical staff standards as defined by comparative data and thresholds, medical literature, and results of peer review evaluations • Use sound clinical judgment based on patient information, available scientific evidence, and patient preferences to develop and carry out patient management plans • Demonstrate caring and respectful behaviors when interacting with patients and their families	• Risk-adjusted mortality by medical diagnosis-related group (DRG) • Risk-adjusted complications by surgical DRG • Peer review cases that are rated inappropriate • Blood transfusions that do not meet established criteria • Percentage of women that had mammogram within the year

 © 2011 HCPro, Inc.

FIGURE 2.2

THE AMERICAN COLLEGE OF PHYSICIAN EXECUTIVES/THE GREELEY COMPANY COMPETENCY FRAMEWORK

Competency area	Demonstration of competency
Technical quality	How specific clinical privileges and general medical skills are used
Service quality	How well communication and response to needs are
Patient safety/rights	How well patients are protected
Resource use	How clinically efficient is utilization of resources
Relationships	How well colleagues and patients are treated
Citizenship	How well medical staff responsibilities are met

Key Considerations for an OPPE Policy

Beyond credentialing, OPPE ensures medical staff quality. Without realizing it, many organizations already perform OPPE to an extent through various practitioner programs. As demonstrated in Figure 2.3, a robust medical staff quality program is made up of a combination of metrics and components from credentialing and privileging processes, peer review metrics, employment contracts, and existing pay-for-performance initiatives. In fact, there is nothing in the regulatory standards that requires that the OPPE process be entirely based on a report. Instead, the standards require that each practitioner be subject to review. There is no reason why OPPE task forces cannot leverage these other quality initiatives and include them in the OPPE program. The key is to organize the components of these typically misaligned initiatives into a formal OPPE process. Integrate physician practice evaluation by merging aspects of OPPE and peer review. This merger is essential because OPPE is, in fact, peer review.

FIGURE 2.3
PROCESSES THAT ALIGN WITH OPPE

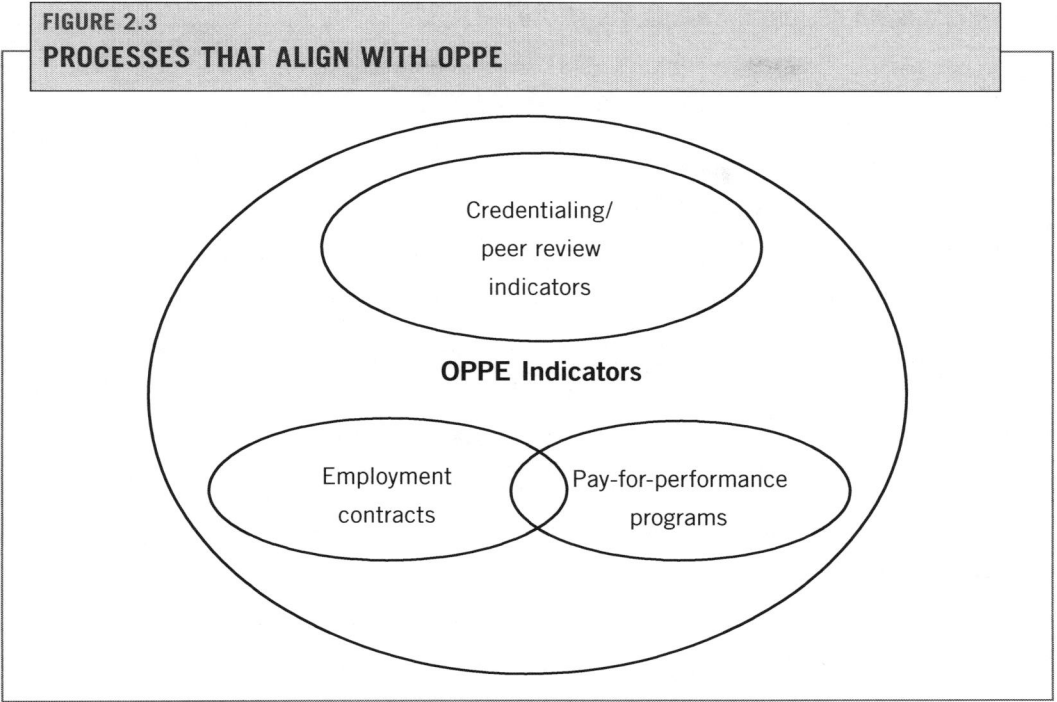

Many organizations have separate policies and procedures for privileging, focused professional practice evaluation (FPPE), OPPE, and peer review, making it appear that each function stands alone or operates independently. This misperception can fragment the competency management program, and participants may have difficulty understanding how all of the elements work together.

There are no rules as to how an organization should structure the overarching process. Medical staffs are free to develop policies that fit their culture and capabilities. Refining the processes will better prepare practitioners to comply with increasingly intense quality mandates from regulators. Quality-oriented medical staff processes are the keys to positioning an organization and its medical staff toward sustainability in a value-driven environment.

 © 2011 HCPro, Inc.

Addressing the medical staff culture

When drafting an OPPE policy, the OPPE task force needs to consider several factors, such as medical staff culture and community norms and how to include physician champions in policy development.

Establishing policies for physician practice evaluation is impossible without addressing the medical staff culture and political issues that may exist. What may seem to be an unequivocal task, such as establishing indicators for review, can have significant repercussions for practitioners who may be concerned about retaining privileges, maintaining a large enough practice base, and their position within the medical staff. Practitioners who see their volume decreasing may be hesitant to establish specific volume thresholds as they may not be able to meet those thresholds one day. Addressing transparency issues regarding physician performance improvement and peer review can be controversial. Although most physicians are now less resistant to discussing data and data sharing, many are still concerned about how their quality information is measured, applied, and shared.

For any organization, developing an overall peer review policy involves researching what other organizations in the community are doing, soliciting feedback from physicians, and communicating the benefits to key stakeholders. Practitioners are often affiliated with more than one hospital in the community and are able to draw from their experiences at those facilities to help develop a peer review policy.

The OPPE task force should solicit the help of a small group of committed physician champions to spearhead the effort and share the policies with the broader medical staff. This group of physician champions should ensure that the goal of providing high quality care and patient safety remains the focus of the effort. Doing so will center the discussion and address both the organization's and practitioners' concerns.

The OPPE task force will likely have to address other elements of an organization's peer review program in the course of developing an OPPE policy. The task force may have to adjust evaluation systems to:

- Ensure a clear understanding of privileging, OPPE, FPPE, and peer review processes and their distinct features and relationships

- Develop new tools to support all phases of practitioner practice evaluation

- Determine where all phases of practice evaluation fit within the existing governance structure of the medical staff

- Determine if aspects of the existing governance structure will require changes to support the processes

Remember, if revisions to these processes are needed to facilitate implementation of a new OPPE process, medical staffs will not have to make changes to the bylaws or governance documents if they are structured so that policies are separate from the governing documents and can be amended with a vote of the medical executive committee (MEC). However, they may require the redefinition of existing committee membership, function, and charters, and/or changes in policies to support practice.

Defining the Scope of the OPPE Program

The OPPE policy should describe the scope of the program and how it will be conducted and supported. When drafting the OPPE policy, medical staffs should answer the following questions:

- How will indicators, data sets, and report production be maintained on an ongoing basis? How will indicators be selected, tested, delivered, and retired?

- Who will be responsible for reviewing the data? This book recommends a triage approach using different levels of reviews involving support staff, such as analysts and clinical staff from either the quality department or medical staff services department and medical staff members and leaders. The more complex the review process is and the greater the number of reviewers there are, the more difficult it may be to maintain protection under the peer review statutes. Another issue to consider when enlisting reviewers of OPPE data is the identification and mitigation of conflicts of interest such as competing practitioners.

- How often will the data be reviewed? Will the data be presented to the practitioner quarterly or every six or nine months? What are the requirements of the relevant accrediting organization? Sharing performance data with physicians annually does not meet The Joint Commission's intent for OPPE. For hospitals that are Joint Commission–accredited, surveyors will consider an annual data-sharing schedule periodic rather than ongoing.

- How will peer review data be used for credentialing and privileging decisions? Do the existing processes support a well-defined procedure for determining whether a physician's privileges should be continued, revised, or revoked?

- Will the data be used to determine quality and safety issues? How will OPPE be integrated with the existing peer review activities and recredentialing?

- Who will make recommendations regarding privileging decisions, and who can take action?

- How are conflicts or dissenting opinions resolved? What are the triggers that raise immediate concerns regarding practitioners' clinical competence? Are the sections of the bylaws that describe activities, such as summary suspension, referenced?

- What will be the process for incorporating OPPE data or results of review into a physician's credentials file? Establish whether OPPE data will be located in the credentials file or whether the credentials file will simply serve as the location for recording results of the review.

- Who can have access to the data? Will access be provided to medical staff leaders, the vice president of medical affairs/chief medical officer? Will organizational administrative staff such as department administrative directors, the chief nursing officer, or the chief operating officer have access?

- How does the OPPE policy link to the FPPE and peer review policies? Will the organization create separate policies for each function, or will it create one umbrella policy that incorporates each of the functions?

The OPPE task force should also consider whether the medical staff governance documents, such as the peer review policy, define processes that support various OPPE outcomes. The task force should look at language in their policies regarding the following processes:

- **Recommendation that a provider continue to exercise the privileges granted.** The peer review committee typically makes this recommendation when a provider performs within the desired thresholds established by the medical staff.

- **Revocation or automatic loss of privilege(s).** The medical staff leadership may determine that a low-volume provider no longer needs a privilege or group of privileges because he or she no longer performs the procedure at the hospital, or because his or her practice has changed and there is insufficient information available to assess clinical competence. In these cases, the privilege may be unilaterally withdrawn with the caveat that in order to reinstitute the privilege, the provider must request the privilege and meet all required documentation to support the request.

- **Referral for FPPE.** If the results of OPPE raise concerns about clinical competence or performance, the medical staff may recommend that a provider undergo FPPE to pinpoint the performance problem.

Once the medical staff answers all of these questions and considers how it will connect the OPPE policy to the organization's overall peer review policy, it's time to start drafting.

Outlining the OPPE Policy

Every OPPE policy should contain the following elements:

1. **Purpose.** The policy should state the reasons for conducting an OPPE and include a description of how the OPPE is integrated into the organization's larger peer review policy. Although the OPPE policy does not have to reference regulatory requirements, it should explain that OPPE is simply another process to assess and ensure competence as a part of the organization's ongoing commitment to a robust quality infrastructure.

2. **Scope and methods of operation.** The scope defines who is responsible for complying with the OPPE policy and procedures, reflects the organization's requirements, and is compatible with the medical staff bylaws or rules and regulations. Consider defining who is subject to the OPPE, the frequency with which OPPE is carried out, the

OPPE framework, the use of the OPPE in decisions regarding providers' privileges, and where results of the OPPE are reported and outcomes are documented.

3.   **Definitions.** Providing definitions of terms used throughout the OPPE policy will help providers speak the same language.

4.   **Goals of the program.** The policy should address the principles on which it is developed and the medical staff's ethical positions on issues such as conflict of interest. The language of the goals should be patient-focused and identify anticipated clinical quality improvement benefits.

5.   **Triggers requiring review.** The policy should outline triggers for FPPE.

6.   **Medical staff oversight.** Identify medical staff members or committees that will have primary oversight for the OPPE process. Individuals who may review OPPE data include the chief medical officer/vice president of medical affairs, clinical service chairs/department chairs/section heads, or other medical staff leaders. Additional levels of review may include the service line or department committees, the medical executive committee (MEC), credentials committee, the quality improvement department, the medical staff services department, and external review organizations. Keep in mind that not every OPPE report must be reviewed. A report may trigger direct evaluation if the results fall below expected thresholds. Describe the integration of the FPPE and peer review processes with the OPPE process and the link to clinical privileging. Establish which committees will be responsible for overseeing the integration of the components and who can make recommendations and take action.

7.   **Authority and responsibilities.** The OPPE policy should spell out the authority and responsibilities regarding the following:

– Creation of the OPPE program

– Accountability for data collection

– Assignment of a group to analyze data and make recommendations

– Policy review and revision

8. **Procedure.** The OPPE report should define what data will be collected, how it will be collected, and how much data is required before the peer review committee can make an informed decision or recommendation regarding a provider's competence. The policy should also define procedures that should be followed when there is insufficient data for evaluation.

9. **Reporting.** The policy should address how and when the data is shared with the provider. It should define the methodology for review and any reporting to medical staff committees.

Ensuring OPPE Program Effectiveness

Once the OPPE program is fully designed and implemented, an oversight committee must oversee it to ensure that the various steps of the process occur as expected and that providers adhere to the procedures. An ineffective (but common) approach to program oversight is having the OPPE, peer review, or credentials committee review all OPPE reports. This approach duplicates the work of medical staff leaders, who have already reviewed OPPE reports. It is far more effective for the dedicated clinical staff to manage the review process at the departmental level and assist the division/section and departmental leaders to ensure that the OPPE process is carried out accordingly.

A best practice is for the OPPE oversight committee to focus its efforts on the following:

- Periodically performing sample audits of each specialty's or department's activities to ensure compliance with procedures

- Assessing whether the OPPE program is providing effective, relevant, and meaningful support for the evaluation of ongoing clinical competence

- Recommending modifications in program configuration, procedures, and training of participants who might improve the effectiveness or efficiency of the program

Many organizations discretely forward results of the OPPE review to the MEC and/or board of directors. Although the MEC and board of directors may need to know individual OPPE results when a privileging action is required, it is not productive to forward detailed results to them. In their capacity as a governing body, the MEC and board of directors are most concerned with ensuring that there are effective systems in place to measure and monitor clinical competence and that there are criteria outlining what should occur when further review or action is needed. The MEC and board of directors should receive periodic reports from the OPPE oversight committee regarding the results of their assessment of the efficiency and effectiveness of the program.

Future revision to the OPPE program, policies, and procedures

Keep in mind that any future revisions to the OPPE policy and procedure will affect the overall peer review program and may affect program operations. The OPPE task force should develop a process for evaluating proposed modifications to determine whether it is worthy of further development and implementation. A review process needs to occur no matter who proposes the modification—a credentialing staff member or the president of the medical staff. This evaluation process is not intended to obstruct continuous improvement,

© 2011 HCPro, Inc. **33**

but rather to provide a mechanism for servicing requests and supporting the deliberate and controlled introduction of improvements.

The evaluation should include a rationale for the proposed modification as well as a description of the following:

- The potential effect the modification will have on resource utilization

- The potential effect the modification will have on work flow and software utilization

- The potential effect the modification will have on quality and timeliness of work products

- The potential revisions that will have to be made to the medical staff bylaws, rules, or regulations if the modification is implemented

- The potential implementation requirements or considerations

Figure 2.4 is a sample proposal that outlines the key considerations the OPPE oversight committee should address.

FIGURE 2.4

SAMPLE MODIFICATIONS TO PEER REVIEW PROGRAM PROPOSAL

1. Explanatory statement or rationale for proposed modification, including anticipated benefits.

2. Potential effect on work flow and software utilization/set up.

3. Potential effect on resource utilization.

4. Potential effect on quality and timeliness of work products.

5. Unanticipated effects if the modification is implemented.

6. Required modifications to medical staff bylaws or rules and regulations (if any).

7. Identification of additional implementation requirements or considerations (timing, training, concurrent projects).

Recommendation to deny proposal:

_____

_____

Recommendation to proceed with the following modifications:

_____

_____

Recommendation to proceed:

_____

_____

| _____ | _____ |
| Authorized signature | Date |

Developing an OPPE Communication Plan

The first time practitioners receive an OPPE report should not be the first time they hear about the program. Ideally, medical staff leaders should inform the general medical staff of the OPPE process from the beginning, whether they are building a new program or revamping an existing one. When medical staff leaders deliver a consistent message about the rationale for OPPE and address the benefits of the program for individual practitioners' perspective, it helps to proactively manage potential pushback from practitioners. In this chapter, we will discuss methods for communicating with and educating practitioners about OPPE.

Creating a Communication Plan

When developing a comprehensive communication plan to educate practitioners on OPPE, use the five W's (who, what, when, where, and why) as a framework to structure your plan:

- Who needs to be educated on OPPE and who will provide that education?

- Why do they need to be educated?

- What information do practitioners need? What are the key messages that need to be conveyed?

- Where should the education on OPPE take place?

- When should practitioners be educated on OPPE?

Who needs to be educated on OPPE and who will provide training?

The OPPE task force should educate key stakeholders, such as medical staff leaders and privileged practitioners on OPPE. It is important that medical staff leaders are on board with OPPE so they can serve as champions of the effort. In addition, medical staff leaders must know what is expected of them during the OPPE process, particularly individuals directly responsible for evaluating the reports.

Educate the following individuals about the OPPE process:

- Medical executive committee (MEC), which will likely include the chief of staff and department/service line chairs

- Credentialing committee

- Peer review committees

- Utilization review committee

- Quality committee

- Other physician-led committees or working groups with physician participants

- Chief nursing officer and/or interdisciplinary practice committee

- In-house counsel and administration

If your hospital pilot tests reports with members of the medical staff, the OPPE task force should communicate the intent of OPPE to them before reaching out to them for pilot testing.

Although the message communicated is important, the messenger is sometimes even more crucial. Any communication regarding OPPE should come from a respected medical staff leader, regardless of whether it is in person or via e-mail. Messages delivered by medical staff leaders promote the leaders' ownership of the program and give the program greater credibility.

Additionally, because OPPE is a medical staff–led program, a message from an appointed or elected medical staff leader will carry far more weight than if it comes from administrative personnel. The messenger that the medical staff chooses varies. The following are a few for consideration:

- Chief medical officer (CMO)/vice president of medical affairs (VPMA)

- Chief of staff (or chief of medicine or surgery)

- Directors of practitioner groups, such as hospitalist leaders

- Department/service line chairs

 © 2011 HCPro, Inc.

What information do practitioners need? What are the key messages that need to be conveyed?

An effective message regarding OPPE should start with the fact that OPPE is a practitioner-led endeavor. When practitioners receive OPPE reports, the first question that comes to mind is: "Why am I receiving this report?" If the medical staff does not proactively answer this question, practitioners will likely come to their own conclusions, and those conclusions may not always be positive or accurate. For example, they might assume that the hospital is monitoring performance for economic purposes. As such, it is important for the medical staff to communicate the reasons for OPPE in a clear and concise manner prior to distributing reports.

Although it may be true that The Joint Commission requires hospitals to evaluate practitioners on an ongoing basis, communicating this as the rationale for the OPPE program may not sufficiently engage practitioners in performance improvement. It may be the technically correct message but it may not be an effective message to engage practitioners as it does not directly impact them. Instead of only answering the question, "What is OPPE?" medical staff leaders should also answer, "Why is understanding individual performance important to both the practitioner and the hospital?"

The following are sample key messages. Consider which of these messages will most appeal to practitioners within your organization:

- OPPE is a medical staff–led initiative to establish performance expectations and ensure that patient care meets expected standards. This should be the constant message in any OPPE communication plan: it is a program by the medical staff for the medical staff.

- Healthcare reform creates the impetus for practitioners to understand their performance data. OPPE allows medical staff to access their own clinical and nonclinical practice data as government proposes new payment structures that are tied to quality of care. The better practitioners understand their performance data, the better they can manage their professional careers within the context of hospital, payer, and patient relationships.

- Healthcare transparency is a growing trend among payers, regulators, and patients. Insurance companies encourage patients to make educated decisions when choosing practitioners by showing practitioner ratings directly on their websites. Regulators make practitioner performance data readily available through programs such as the Centers for Medicare & Medicaid Services (CMS) Physician Compare website. Patients proactively research practitioners and hospitals using resources such as UCompare (*www.ucompare.com*) and HealthGrades (*www.healthgrades.com*). OPPE gives practitioners similar visibility into their own performance data.

- Hospital/medical staff partnerships allow administrators and practitioners to come together to understand and act on opportunities to improve the quality of patient care. OPPE provides the vehicle for this collaboration.

- Professional development opportunities occur when practitioners compare their performance against that of their peers. OPPE gives practitioners access to timely data that allows them to further their career growth by improving performance in key areas deemed significant to their practice.

- Organizational quality goals and initiatives should be included in every medical staff's OPPE communication plan. OPPE can be a vehicle for organizations to implement these initiatives for individual practitioners.

Once medical staff leaders develop the broader message regarding OPPE, that message should guide the content of all communication. Create a more detailed message to those leaders who participate in developing the OPPE process, whether they help select indicators or thresholds or review and evaluate practitioners.

Consider the culture of the medical staff when creating the OPPE communication plan. Avoid using language or phrases that strike a nerve with the medical staff. Doing so will distract from the message being conveyed. Although the specific terms practitioners find offensive may vary by culture, some examples that may have negative connotations are as follows:

- Economic credentialing

- Physician profiling

- Physician performance management

- Physician cost reduction

- Practitioner grade

Where should the education on OPPE take place?

Medical staffs congregate for a variety of meetings throughout the year. Take advantage of these opportunities to educate practitioners on OPPE. The greatest benefit of in-person meetings is that they provide a forum for questions, feedback, and suggestions. If these meetings are well attended, you can reach a broad audience; however, this may not always be the case. Some hospitals organize enticing dinners or offer continuing medical education credits to encourage providers to participate in meetings. Even if such enticements are successful, medical staff leaders are unlikely to reach 100% of practitioners, so it's important to use multiple modes of communication, such as:

- Newsletter articles

- E-mail memos

- Traditional mailed letters/memos

- Automated voice mail

- Individual conversations between medical staff leaders and practitioners

These indirect forms of communication allow medical staff leaders to broadly disseminate a well-crafted message. Unfortunately, medical staff leaders always run the risk of such messages being ignored. It is best to include both direct and indirect forms of communication in your plan to ensure that practitioners hear and remember the message. Because each person learns differently (some people are visual learners and some are more auditory) medical staff leaders should deliver key messages and education more than once and via more than one approach.

When should practitioners be educated on OPPE?

OPPE reports should not catch practitioners by surprise. Create a timeline around which all practitioners will receive OPPE education, particularly if the medical staff is adopting a new reporting process.

In addition to the initial education, consider strategies for longer term communication, which could likely include the same venues and modes of communication. Figure 3.1 is a sample communication plan, which should be an ever-growing document. It includes multiple modes of communication and reiteration of the message through different venues. Once initial communication is complete, keep the forum open to allow the medical staff to communicate updates to the OPPE process and allow practitioners to provide feedback.

FIGURE 3.1

SAMPLE OPPE COMMUNICATION PLAN

Audience	Purpose	Forum	Date/time	Messenger	Additional targeted messages
MEC	Educate on the OPPE requirement and engage participation in indicator/threshold selection process	MEC meeting		CMO	MEC will need to authorize the OPPE program and the medical staff leaders will be responsible for evaluating OPPE reports every six months
Surgery department	General OPPE education	Surgery department meeting		Chief of surgery	

Preparing for Pushback

No matter how much work the OPPE task force does or how solid the OPPE program appears, it is likely that some practitioners will push back. Some complaints may be legitimate and will require the OPPE task force to go back to the drawing board.

Other complaints may come from practitioners who are unwilling to change. Often, these practitioners misunderstand the intent of the OPPE program. Take the time to craft thoughtful responses to the following common concerns that practitioners often express:

- Is OPPE a way for hospitals to control how practitioners practice medicine?

- Is OPPE a way to "punish" high-cost practitioners?

- Is my OPPE data used by my competitors to control or stifle my practice?

- Will outlier performance result in an immediate loss of privileges?

- Is the medical staff rolling out OPPE simply to comply with Joint Commission regulations?

- Are practitioner concerns considered? Are practitioners even included in the decision-making process?

- The data are wrong so the reports are worthless.

Proactively addressing these questions in a nonhostile manner will be much easier than reacting to them. Head off some of these concerns by emphasizing the following points in all communication materials:

- **OPPE is a practitioner-led program.** Medical staff leaders are ultimately responsible for selecting indicators and thresholds by specialty. Each clinical department should be involved in the design of the OPPE approach for its specialty. The MEC approves the approach and the policy. Administration's role is to support the medical staff.

- **Indicators.** If cost indicators are used, the medical staff must clearly embrace them as a legitimate indicator or factor in quality of care. Although it is true that OPPE will identify practitioners who fall short on performance, OPPE's ultimate goal is to affirm clinical competence, support practitioners, and help them improve performance. Just because a practitioner's performance falls below thresholds does not necessarily mean that the medical staff will take action against his or her privileges. The first step is to validate a practitioner's outlier status by doing a case-level analysis to confirm that practitioners' concerns are warranted.

- **The purpose of OPPE.** Although OPPE is a requirement for Joint Commission–accredited hospitals, the primary purpose of OPPE is to achieve clinical excellence and is thus considered a best practice for all hospitals, regardless of which accreditation agency they use. Always bring the rationale for performance improvement back to the key messages the organization identified when it designed its OPPE communication plan.

- **Data concerns.** Although OPPE data should undergo stringent tests to ensure that it is as accurate as possible, the OPPE task force should investigate all concerns that practitioners bring to its attention and resolve any valid issues. Medical staff leaders should remind practitioners that imperfect data are still valuable information; it sheds light on data errors that must be fixed, especially is this data is used by payers to determine incentives. Data-driven performance measurements are here to stay—we need to master them.

- **Attribution (case assignment).** The attribution policy and process can be a huge area of contention for practitioners. One of the biggest challenges with OPPE is the process of assigning one physician to a patient, when in reality there are multiple practitioners providing care. The key to addressing this risk is to proactively understand the current process and standardize attribution inconsistencies to create the most accurate process for your organization.

- **Misaligned physician documentation and abstraction/coding.** Inappropriate documentation (both under- and over-documentation) can lead to inaccurate abstraction or coding, which affects severity adjustment and the accuracy of indicators derived from codes. Undercoding can result in imprecise severity comparisons. For example, if respiratory failure patients are coded as pneumonia patients because comorbidities are not documented, it will appear that patient outcomes are worse than expected because pneumonia patients typically have lower expected mortality rates. If imprecise documentation results in expected conditions as being coded as complications, a practitioner's complication rates could be higher than average. For example, overall complication rates will be affected if postop ileus is tagged as a complication in major large and small bowel procedures although the practitioner did not mean for it to be tagged as a complication. Just like with attribution challenges, it is important to take a proactive approach to streamlining documentation and coding. Many hospitals have complications policies and documentation improvement programs in place to help reduce miscommunications between practitioners and coders. Clinical documentation specialists are also helpful resources to train practitioners on little known facts (i.e., nursing documentation should not be used for coding). If providers have concerns around coding, be prepared to explain the relationship between coding and documentation and the efforts the hospital is making to help mitigate problems.

- **Competing priorities.** Practitioners are often pulled in multiple directions. Assess what other projects require practitioners' time to ensure that OPPE does not become overwhelming in light of other projects. If practitioners are clearly overloaded, the organization may need to reprioritize the demands placed on them and table or streamline quality improvement activities so that practitioner participation in the most important initiatives is thoughtful, meaningful, and beneficial to the practitioner, their patients, and to the organization.

Selecting Data for the OPPE Program

Understanding
Performance Indicators

Selecting performance indicators is one of the most important responsibilities an OPPE task force will need to complete. Performance indicators are the heart of OPPE data, and thoughtfully and carefully selecting the best indicators is crucial to obtaining meaningful and reliable data.

This chapter focuses on the following topics:

- Understanding the three types of indicators: rate, rule, and review

- Formulating a multiphase project plan for selecting and implementing indicators based on data availability, development work effort, and the organization's competency framework

- Creating an inventory of potential indicators from internal and external resources

- Testing the validity and integrity of potential indicators

- Selecting nonclinical and clinical indicators and engaging practitioners in the process

- Creating an indicator implementation work plan with a manageable timeline

- Managing the demand for desirable yet unavailable indicators

- Not waiting for perfection

Types of Indicators: Rate, Rule, and Review

Before delving into a discussion regarding indicator selection, it is important to understand the difference between the three types of indicators: review, rule, and rate. Knowing how the indicators differ helps you determine the data elements needed to calculate each indicator and the level of analysis necessary should the indicator raise a red flag as the type of indicator is indicative of performance expectations and risk potential.

Review indicators

Review indicators flag serious or complex events that require further analysis to determine cause, effect, and severity. These are traditional peer review cases whereby any violation triggers a chart review. Examples include actual reports of harm to a patient or potentially adverse events (near misses), patient safety indicators (PSI), and perioperative/procedural mortality.

Rule indicators

Rule indicators represent a standard, generally recognized professional guideline or a practice wherein individual variation does not directly cause adverse patient outcomes. Rule indicators focus on conformance with recognized best practices. Rule indicators identify how many times a practitioner's performance falls outside accepted standards, or where perfect compliance is a reasonable expectation but some degree of variation does not

 © 2011 HCPro, Inc.

necessarily indicate a problem. They are typically expressed in terms of the number of permissible violations. For example, the medical staff may require practitioners to partici- pate in a preprocedure "timeout." Practitioners who never break this rule (zero incidents) might be considered excellent performers in this area. The medical staff may consider two or fewer incidents in a one-year period as an acceptable level of performance, but any more incidents might be considered unacceptable and trigger additional follow-up.

A criticism of rule indicators is that they do not take into account a practitioner's volume of activity and are thus biased against high-volume practitioners. Therefore, when appropriate and when denominator volumes are available, use rate indicators instead of rule indicators. Rate indicators level the playing field by adjusting for volume. However, use rule indicators to prevent a practitioner's volume of work from being an excuse for failing to comply.

Rate indicators

Rate indicators measure the frequency of an expected event, typically expressed as a percentage, percentile rank, average, or ratio. This means that rate indicators require a numerator and a denominator for calculation. Often, perfect compliance is not a reason- able expectation, which is why expressing results as a percentage or ratio of relevant cases makes more sense than a hard number. Examples include complication rates, core measures compliance, and readmission rates, which measure how often an expected event does or does not occur.

Rate indicators have the following advantages:

- They allow for easy statistical analysis and severity/acuity adjustment.

- They are more efficient than review indicators because they do not require individual chart reviews for every outlying case.

© 2011 HCPro, Inc. **53**

- They allow for acceptable variations within the context of patient volumes. For example, perforations during colonoscopies occur even with the most experienced and skilled gastroenterologists. Examining each case individually is unnecessary and an inefficient use of time. Instead, compare a practitioner's perforation rates (such as the percentage of perforations) with peers performing the same procedure, regardless of volume.

Rate indicators have the following limitations:

- Not all indicators will have denominators, making it impossible to calculate a rate indicator.

- Processes performed infrequently will have low denominators, thus any change in the numerator (the number of successes or failures) is exaggerated, and the data are deemed statistically unreliable. One solution to this situation is to use a longer time frame or to use a rule indicator.

Developing a Plan for Selecting Indicators and Gathering Data

Every organization is at a different point in developing its OPPE program. A multistep approach to creating the OPPE program and selecting indicators allows the OPPE task force to tailor the process to its unique work stream and needs. The project planning approach will depend on whether the organization currently produces OPPE or practitioner feedback reports. The following are two examples of phased approaches to selecting indicators or enriching existing OPPE reports with new indicators. In both approaches, it is important to note that the OPPE task force is responsible for leading and coordinating the OPPE development process with collaborations, assistance, and feedback from medical staff leaders from departments/divisions within the organization.

Example 1: Indicator selection based on data availability and minimal development work effort

The goal of the first approach is to select indicators based on their level of availability and ease of access. The OPPE task force first seeks to leverage existing data collection efforts for the new OPPE program. As the reporting mechanism becomes more robust, the medical staff may choose to introduce more complex indicators that are not as easily available. With the ability to better define indicators and collect data, the hospital can produce data that subspecialists find more relevant to the determination of clinical competence.

The following outlines the four phases of this approach:

- Phase 1: The OPPE task force and medical staff leaders identify readily available indicators that the organization already captures for other reporting purposes, such as core measures and indicators tied to existing employment contracts, pay-for-performance initiatives, and other practitioner programs that track data.

- Phase 2: Facilitate data gathering by making small process changes or updates in technology systems that do not require a lot of time or work effort.

- Phase 3: Put forth additional effort to gather data within current organizational capabilities. This may require more substantial process changes; additional staff, such as IT or administrative; and/or new resources as needed.

- Phase 4: Identify infrastructure enhancements and resources needed to facilitate the collection of data that does not exist for indicators.

 © 2011 HCPro, Inc.

Example 2: Indicator selection based on the competency framework

The second approach to selecting and gathering data for indicators is based on the competency categories within the performance framework.

If the OPPE task force chooses to use the competency framework developed by the American Academy of Physician Executives/Greeley Company, a division of HCPro, Inc., versus the framework developed by Accreditation Council for Graduate Medical Education (ACGME)/American Board of Medical Specialties (ABMS), use the crosswalk in Figure 4.1 to select indicators most applicable to the practitioner, hospital, department, or specialty level.

FIGURE 4.1
COMPETENCY FRAMEWORK CROSSWALK

ACPE/ Greeley	Patient care	Medical knowledge	Practice-based learning	Interpersonal/ communication skills	Professionalism	Systems-based practice
Technical quality	Specialty-specific	Hospital level				
Service quality	Specialty-specific			Hospital level	Hospital level	Department-specific
Patient safety/rights	Specialty-specific			Hospital level	Hospital level	Department-specific
Resource use						Department-specific
Relationships				Hospital level	Hospital level	
Citizenship			Hospital level		Hospital level	

Source: Adapted from The Greeley Company, a division of HCPro, Inc.

 © 2011 HCPro, Inc. THE COMPLETE GUIDE TO OPPE

Phase 1: Choose indicators that apply to all or most practitioners at the organization

Of the six competency areas set forth in the ACGME/ABMS framework, the following typically apply to most practitioners regardless of their specialty or area of practice:

- Medical/clinical knowledge

- Practice-based learning and improvement

- Interpersonal and communication skills

- Professionalism

Initially, focus the organization's OPPE indicators on these areas. Indicators that fall into these competency categories include:

- Peer review cases

- Reported patient and family complaints

- Continuing medical education credits related to specialty or privileges requested

- Board certification requirements

Phase 2: Department-specific indicators

Next, select indicators that apply to specific departments or clinical service areas, such as medicine, surgery, and OB/GYN (most specialties can be grouped into one of these three categories). For example, indicators related to the systems-based practice competency (ACGME/ABMS) apply only to specific groups of physicians. OPPE task forces would select procedural volumes and outcomes as indicators for surgical specialties but not medical specialties.

  © 2011 HCPro, Inc.

Phase 3: Specialty-specific indicators

Select indicators relevant to individual specialties. Remember that OPPE results are factored into decisions to maintain, revise, or revoke privileges at or prior to reappointment, so some of the indicators should relate to the practitioners' clinical specialty.

Selecting indicators across multiple specialties can be a daunting task. Work with small groups of specialties at a time, starting with the easiest ones first, such as inpatient specialties with high volumes, because you will have more data to work with. Additionally, if physicians in two or more specialties provide similar care, such as internal medicine and family practice, consider selecting the same indicators for both specialties because practitioner performance is typically measured using similar indicators.

TIP

Prior to selecting specialty-specific indicators, take the time to verify your specialties from an OPPE perspective. The physician roster typically lists the hospital's specialties and the physicians who practice in each one. Because patient care indicators are selected at the specialty level, you may run into reporting areas if practitioners are not listed in the correct specialty.

Depending on how the medical staff is structured, physician rosters may contain a larger list of specialties than are truly necessary for OPPE. The OPPE task force should consider streamlining and consolidating them for simplicity. The task force may consider grouping the specialties, particularly if care provided by some practitioners spans multiple specialties, or one practitioner leader oversees several overlapping specialties.

OPPE task forces may also choose a hybrid approach, using elements of both methods for selecting indicators. When using the competency framework phased approach, the OPPE task force may also consider rating the indicators based on how much work they require. The task force can prioritize the indicators not only by their applicability to practitioners, but also by the amount of work necessary to develop them.

Once the OPPE task force chooses a philosophy for indicator selection, it must inventory indicators, choose the ones that are best suited for OPPE, evaluate those indicators, and gain approval from the medical staff. The following sections describe each of these activities, and Figure 4.2 is a flow chart depicting the steps OPPE task forces take to select indicators.

FIGURE 4.2
INDICATOR SELECTION FLOW CHART

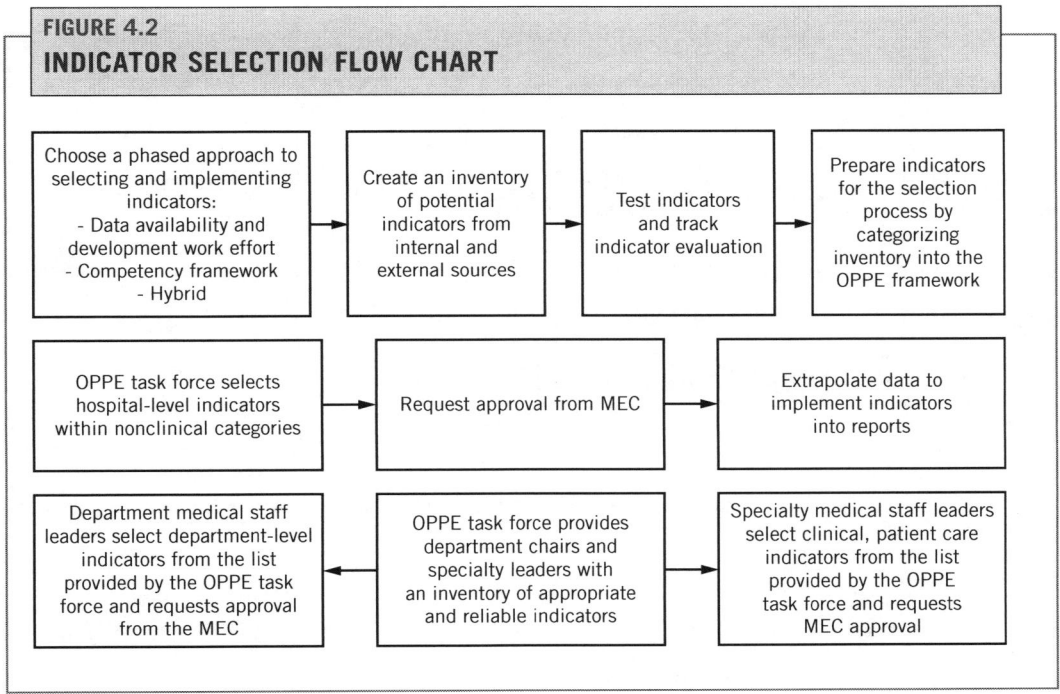

Creating an Inventory of Potential Indicators

Some organizations simply layer new program requirements on top of existing efforts, missing the opportunity to evaluate and streamline the entire clinical quality improvement program. Ensure an efficient OPPE process by creating an inventory of all existing data collection efforts and peer review screens and assessing whether the specific measures are of value to the organization. During this process, also review indicators suggested by external national organizations that are actively involved in clinical performance measurement initiatives and benchmarking. The following section reviews examples of internal and external resources for indicators OPPE task forces may consult when developing their inventories.

Internal resources for indicators

Existing organizational and department initiatives contain a plethora of performance data. The OPPE task force and medical staff leaders from each department should look first at clinical indicators that the medical staff has previously vetted and approved. Examine the data gathered to identify indicators specific to practitioner performance.

The following is a list of common existing clinical and administrative initiatives that often use indicators that may be appropriate to include in the OPPE program:

- Credentialing/privileging reports used for reappointment profiling or decision-making

- Performance mandates included in bylaws, regulations, and other internal policies (e.g., compliance with on-call response)

- Performance mandates or objectives included in the organizational strategic plan, leadership experience, and vision

- Measures or indicators previously identified as part of the organizational quality plan

- Requirements incorporated into existing employment contracts with performance-driven bonus structures

- Indicators or measures incorporated into existing pay-for-performance initiatives and other performance-driven reimbursement payment structures

- Clinical integration and accountable care initiatives (e.g., core measures)

- Compliance measures associated with clinical documentation improvement initiatives

- Lean/Six Sigma programs

- Performance objectives previously identified by specialty-specific task forces and committees

- Peer review screening indicators

- Case review results/scores

- Medical staff services department (e.g., medical malpractice occurrence reports or other external data)

- Surgery and emergency department operational measures (e.g., OR delayed starts due to physician)

- Patient satisfaction surveys

- Other practitioner feedback reports

External resources for indicators

OPPE task forces should make an effort to ensure that OPPE indicators are meaningful, strong enough to impact performance, moving practitioners closer to global evidence-based clinical excellence or best practices based upon peer consensus. With that said, consider including indicators from external resources, such as specialty societies and governmental programs. Report indicators recommended by external organizations or use them as benchmarks for internal performance improvement initiatives.

Many organizations have developed specifications for indicators (e.g., numerators, denominators, and sources) and evaluated their feasibility of collection, validity, relevance, and stability. Many of these organizations benchmark indicators or measures that hospitals already have to report. It's up to the OPPE task force to decide whether it wants to use the data for internal quality improvement activities. The following organizations have defined clinical indicators for practitioner performance measurement:

- The Agency for Healthcare Research and Quality (AHRQ): AHRQ collects and publicly reports quality improvement data at the individual practitioner level across millions of Medicare discharges. This enables organizations to benchmark themselves against other organizations. The AHRQ website contains additional details (*http://www.ahrq.gov/*).

- Centers for Medicare & Medicaid Services (CMS): Because Medicare reimbursement is linked to compliance with best practices and hospitals expend considerable effort to collect and review this performance data, such as core measures and hospitals acquired conditions. It may be beneficial to leverage these efforts into OPPE reporting. Linking core measures to authorization of privileges may help medical staffs emphasize to physicians the importance of complying with best practices. Additionally, CMS has other optional programs beyond core measures that establish practitioner performance expectations across the continuum of care. These additional programs include the collection of data in private practice offices and clinics, as well as hospitals. Data that has already been collected by these programs indicate that problematic management of care across the continuum may affect the reimbursement to all stakeholders within a practice group or hospital. Some noteworthy programs include Practitioner Quality Reporting System (PQRS), formerly known as Practitioner Quality Reporting Initiative (PQRI), and Value-Based Purchasing. Find more information at *https://www.cms.gov/PQRS/* and *http://www.ahrq.gov/qual/meyerrpt.htm.*

- American Medical Association programs: Practitioner Consortium for Performance Improvement fosters quality and patient safety. More information can be found at *http://www.ama-assn.org/ama/pub/physician-resources/clinical-practice-improvement/ clinical-quality/physician-consortium-performance-improvement.page.*

- Proprietary specialty databases: Many organizations participate and report to specialty programs, such as the American College of Cardiology, Society for Thoracic Surgery, National Comprehensive Cancer Network, American Society for Radiation Oncology, National Cardiovascular Data Registry, and CARE Registry for carotid artery revascularization and endarterctomy procedures. If the physicians have already shown interest and placed value in these indicators by subscribing to these databases and the hospital is already devoting resources to abstracting and reporting data, leverage these efforts into the OPPE program.

- National Committee for Quality Assurance

- National Quality Forum Endorsed Measures

- Clinical practice guidelines and clinical pathways

- Institute for Healthcare Improvement

- Patient satisfaction vendor data

- Centers of Excellence (COE): Commercial payers are now requiring access to hospitals' registry data as part of the COE applications. The OPPE task force may wish to include the practitioner-specific measures as part of the OPPE framework.

- Accrediting agencies: Some accreditation organizations now require the delivery of high quality care and the demonstration of quality improvement through disease-specific certifications. Some payers also require that organizations have certified or accredited programs in order to qualify for payment, such as American Society for Bariatric Surgery certification or American College of Surgeons trauma program certification. For accredited hospitals, these certifications are optional. Each of the defined certifications may have measures that can be translated into practitioner-specific indicators.

Narrowing down the list of potential indicators

Once the task force has an inventory of potential indicators from internal and external sources, it should assess the relevance of each indicator and the integrity of available data before incorporating them into the OPPE process. During this process, the OPPE task force can also identify indicators that may improve practitioner performance, patient care, and clinical service. This is not meant to be a comprehensive review of the indicators for selection into the OPPE program. That comes in the next step. Instead, focus on narrowing down this list of data to those most relevant to OPPE.

Once the OPPE task force narrows down the list of available indicators into an inventory potentially relevant to OPPE, it can begin the selecting indicators.

Selecting Nonclinical and Clinical Indicators

The OPPE task force should select hospital-level indicators under the direction of medical staff leaders from each department/division. Ideally, the same medical staff leaders who assisted in creating the indicator inventory will also help the OPPE task force select indicators.

The OPPE task force and medical staff should evaluate the indicators on the inventory, looking at validity, accuracy, benefits, attribution, communicability, competency, and data availability. Use the checklist in Figure 4.3 to evaluate indicators based on these elements.

The type of indicators selected typically correlate to the level of subspecialization of the peer group. The chiefs/chairs of the medicine, surgery, and OB/GYN departments should select indicators within the system-based practice category for their respective departments. The subspecialty chiefs/chairs should select indicators relevant to patient care. Medical staff leaders, such as the medical executive committee (MEC), should approve the selected indicators.

FIGURE 4.3

INDICATOR INTEGRITY CRITERIA CHECKLIST

❏ **Validity:** What is the relevancy of the indicator to practitioner performance? How strong is the scientific evidence supporting the validity of the indicator as a quality measure? Does the indicator measure the aspect of performance it is purported to measure? Consider the example of chest pain patients who are supposed to receive aspirin at arrival (a CMS core measure). At some hospitals, this is the responsibility of the practitioner who has to write an order, whereas at other hospitals, it is delegated to the nursing staff. In the latter instance, the indicator is no longer valid to practitioner performance management because practitioners are not responsible for variances.

❏ **Reliability:** Are the results of the indicator consistent and reproducible? Does the measure provide for fair comparisons of the performance of practitioners, facilities, health plans, or geographic areas?

❏ **Accuracy:** Does the calculation methodology and specifications lead to a result that is close to the actual or true result? Are all individuals in the denominator equally eligible for inclusion in the numerator? An accurate indicator of the quality of care should exclude patients who should not receive the indicated care or are not at risk for the outcome.

❏ **Benefit:** Does the cost of data collection outweigh the performance improvement opportunities? Does the measure directly align with the organization's strategy and performance improvement goals?

❏ **Attribution:** Is the indicator result under the control of an individual practitioner? Can the organization's attribution policy support the inclusion of the measure? For example, an organization's pharmacy and laboratory systems contain valuable data but inaccurate practitioner attribution.

❏ **Communicability:** Can physicians easily understand the definition and rationale for the indicator?

FIGURE 4.3

INDICATOR INTEGRITY CRITERIA CHECKLIST (CONT.)

❏ **Competency:** Does the indicator relate to an important expectation of performance within the OPPE competency framework? If an indicator is relevant but does not fall within the competency framework, does the indicator align with the organization's goals for OPPE? If it does not fall within the performance framework that the organization has selected, the OPPE task force may need to revisit the framework and goals.

❏ **Data availability and development work effort:** How readily can the data be gathered to calculate the indicator? Is the data collection process manageable given possible constraints in organizational resources?

❏ **Data source:** Where should the data come from? Does it come from administrative systems, clinical documentation, coded data, incident reports, perception surveys, or clinical data registries?

Figure 4.4 is an example of an inventory tool that OPPE tasks forces can use to track indicators.

 © 2011 HCPro, Inc.

FIGURE 4.4
SAMPLE INDICATOR SELECTION INVENTORY

Potential indicator	Validity/ practitioner relevancy	Indicator reliability	Calculation accuracy	Benefit to goals	Attribution accuracy	Communicability	Competency category	Work effort	Data source
Maternal death									
Patient falls									
Number of peer review cases									
Patient satisfaction score									
Delayed or first case starts due to surgeon									
Severity-adjusted LOS									
Nonresponsive to on-call ED pages									
Meeting attendance									

Aligning organizational goals with the OPPE initiative

Aligning OPPE indicators with the organization's strategy and priorities is crucial to integrating practitioner performance into the medical staff's broader quality infrastructure and accountability model. Although organizations often attempt to communicate their goals to the medical staff, the message does not always resonate with everyone. Staff assigned to support the development of the OPPE program should consider providing a summarized list of the organizationwide goals and those of each department or specialty. Also encourage physician leaders to keep these goals at hand when selecting indicators. Add context to the goals by sharing information regarding current performance and areas needing improvement on the medical staff, department, or individual practitioner level. Tying indicators to potential or actual performance issues or variability among practitioners is a great way to encourage targeted improvements.

Use goal cascading to operationalize the indicator selection process. Goal cascading is the concept of linking business goals and performance measures to individual performance targets. This concept can be applied to OPPE. Identify relevant organizational and department/specialty goals and link them to performance indicators that measure how successfully a practitioner performs within the context of the organization's goals. This process shows the specific effect a physician's performance has on the specialty, department, and entire hospital.

With goal cascading, the OPPE task force can effectively bridge the organizational goals and OPPE indicators into a robust quality infrastructure. Ideally, OPPE will function as a vehicle for achieving goals, and practitioners will clearly understand the effect of their performance on the hospital's strategy.

How many indicators are appropriate?

The Joint Commission has not provided a strict standard regarding the number of indicators organizations should select for an OPPE program. Fewer than five indicators may not provide a balanced view of the practitioner's performance, but more than 20 indicators will most likely require a significant investment of resources to capture and analyze the data.

Initially, the OPPE task force may select only one indicator per competency category. This allows the task force to determine whether the resulting report can be produced with existing resources and whether attribution issues have been addressed. Taking this approach will assist in achieving early success with the program, attaining program credibility and gaining momentum for future efforts.

As the program evolves, the organization may consider selecting two to three indicators per competency category, resulting in 12 to 18 indicators practitioners can use to manage their performance. Selecting a manageable number of indicators should make it easier for the OPPE task force to gain the support of the medical staff and work through any issues that may surface while rolling out the OPPE program. Although the OPPE task force may have to start with a smaller number of indicators, having 12 to 18 indicators provides a balanced view of a practitioner's performance and highlights patterns and trends for review.

Additionally, a manageable number of indicators reduces the chance that practitioners will be overwhelmed by the data and will ignore OPPE reports. It is far more important to select a few indicators that are relevant to clinical practice and to meet requirements for validity, specificity, and data integrity than it is to offer numerous indicators that lack relevance or data integrity. As the OPPE process matures, the medical staff will most likely add more indicators. Prevent the proliferation of indicators by retiring existing indicators as new ones are added.

Because clinical patient care indicators are specialty-specific, the OPPE task force will have a large amount of data to capture and organize. Indicators must be measurable, meaningful, linked to organizational performance improvement priorities, and useful in making decisions regarding renewal of privileges. Quality is better than quantity in this situation, so resist the urge to include indicators just because they are easy to collect and/or report.

TIP

Organizational priorities are constantly evolving. Organizations should inventory all existing data collection efforts and peer review screens related to competency management and confirm whether the specific measures are yielding value to the organization. As medical staff leaders identify initiatives, add new indicators to the OPPE program. Retiring indicators that no longer provide value or have not presented opportunities for improvement frees up department resources to assist with new initiatives or new requests for data and will refresh efforts as OPPE reports are designed and implemented. As medical staff leaders identify new measures/indicators, update the data collection work plan.

Tracking Indicator Implementation With a Data Collection Work Plan

As the OPPE task force and medical staff leaders go through the process of selecting indicators, maintain a data collection work plan to track implementation efforts of approved indicators. During the selection process, the OPPE task force should evaluate data availability and document the work effort that collecting the data will entail in the Indicator Selection Inventory. The OPPE task force can expand this inventory to also indicate and track other information, such as:

- Priority: Indicate which indicators the task force will focus on first

- Ownership: Define who is responsible for gathering the data

The data collection work plan also requires the OPPE task force to define specifications for the indicators, including numerators and denominators, adjustments to the data (i.e., excluded populations), attribution of the indicator, and any known limitations of the indicator. The plan recognizes anticipated data integrity problems up front so that users can decide if they are comfortable with identified defects or if they would like to reject or further modify proposed measures. During these discussions, the task force should identify possible performance ranges and thresholds or triggers for each indicator that may signal potentially adverse findings.

DOWNLOADABLE TOOL

Download a sample data collection work plan by visiting the link provided at the beginning of this book.

Plan for the long term by developing a quality control plan that outlines the frequency with which the indicator will be delivered so that data owners are aware of the expectations. Do not be surprised if the OPPE program and data collection become a long-term project. Having a one- or two-year work plan is better than inadvertently dropping indicators from the list or setting unattainable expectations that require substantial rework, insufficient buy-in from key stakeholders, and/or a loss of program credibility. The keys to success are a clearly defined project structure and clearly assigned roles in the project. As such, the OPPE task force should proactively define who is responsible for specific tasks and set timelines based on work effort, available resources, and the significance of indicators to help

 © 2011 HCPro, Inc.

the organization reach its immediate OPPE goals. Set specific goals and review progress quarterly, update priorities, and recognize or elevate incomplete activities in order to get back on track. Without a tightly managed project plan and timeline, executive support, and accountability structure, failure is a certainty.

A Warning on Waiting for Perfection

Searching for perfect indicators may be futile. Although some indicators are great to have, the OPPE task force may not have the necessary data to create the desired indicators, or the indicators might require extensive resources to collect. This is why we suggest creating an inventory of readily available and reliable indicators. During the indicator selection process, if the OPPE task force runs into a popular measurement that is simply not available, create a wish list of potential indicators to be captured in the future. This gives the task force the opportunity to vet and test the indicator, and determine the source, attribution, and feasibility prior to deploying it. However, do not let this be a bottleneck in the process of selecting indicators and do not get stuck on one indicator. Select from what is feasible and currently available while the OPPE task force decides on whether to invest the time and resources required to create an indicator for future use. The following questions will help with that decision:

- What is the end goal of this popular yet unavailable measurement?

- What is the anticipated impact on quality of care?

- Does the measurement fall within the organization's goals and competency framework?

- Is it crucial to the success of the practitioners' performance improvement and the OPPE program?

© 2011 HCPro, Inc.

- Is there another indicator that might help achieve this same goal or measure the same or similar activity or process? If there is, be realistic about using more accessible indicators.

- Does the benefit of creating this indicator outweigh the work effort (time and resources) needed?

If the final decision is that this new measurement is worth pursuing, be prescriptive about the data capture process. Include this indicator in the data collection work plan only if the OPPE task force can answer the following questions:

- Are the data needed to calculate this indicator captured in an electronic system?

- If so, who can extract the data? If not, how will the data be captured?

- Who will be responsible for capturing the data?

- In what format would the OPPE task force need the data, and what is the timeline?

If there are multiple indicators that need to be captured manually, consider using one document to capture the data. A spreadsheet or database is typically a better choice than a word processing document, so that the data can be manipulated more effectively.

DOWNLOADABLE TOOL

A sample spreadsheet capturing several manual indicators is included the downloadable materials that accompany this book.

Using Perception Data as a Source for OPPE Evaluations

Perception data differ from clinical data in that they are based on how others view a practitioner's performance in relatively subjective areas. Interpersonal and communication skills and professionalism competencies are best measured through reported observations (negative or positive) by peers, coworkers, supervisors, and patients. This is called perception data. Incident reports, such as complaints and compliments, are single-event perception data.

The use of perception data to evaluate practitioners is not a new concept. Residency programs first emphasized the importance of aggregate perception data, particularly by including the opinions of nonphysicians in performance evaluations. For practicing physicians, this is still a fairly new concept. Using others' views about practitioners' behavior will likely create some unease and potentially overt hostility for those who are not accustomed to it. As such, it is important to understand how best to obtain perception data and how to introduce their use to the medical staff.

Perception data help practitioners understand how others perceive their actions, regardless of their intentions. Although a practitioner might think that he or she is communicating clearly to a patient, it is really the patient's perception of the clarity of the message that

© 2011 HCPro, Inc.

counts. For example, a practitioner might discuss potential complications of a procedure in precise technical language with a patient who has no clinical background and is too intimidated or simply not comfortable asking questions. The practitioner may leave the room feeling the conversation went well. The patient, however, may have a different perspective.

When Should Perception Data Be Used?

Hospitals can best use perception data to evaluate performance-related expectations for the following:

- Interpersonal relationship skills

- Communication

- Professionalism

- Social interactions or team cooperation

- Oral and written communication skills

- Responsiveness

- Sensitivity to diversity

Consider the following scenario using a physician's responsiveness as an example of perception data. Many organizations have a specific standard defining the expected response time for an emergency department (ED) or obstetrical call. Others may specify an expected time frame in which an attending is expected to respond to calls regarding inpatients under his or her supervision. The medical staff bylaws, rules and regulations, and/or policies typically outline these expectations. Most organizations do not actively track compliance with these expectations. Instead, they enforce the requirement by exception.

For example, when staff members report that a practitioner did not respond in a timely manner to an ED call, the practitioner may receive a letter or phone call from the department chair emphasizing the necessity to comply with the requirement. This approach to data collection is considered passive because the medical staff does not solicit this information. These types of events and their subsequent intervention may be recorded and scored as a peer-reviewed case and may appear on the OPPE report under the "case review" section as a separate event or occurrence. Hospitals may also use perception data when objective data are not available or are difficult to collect. For example, there may not be an effective way to evaluate practitioners' professionalism with colleagues other than using complaint incident reports.

Alternatively, organizations may elect to actively collect perception data. The medical staff could send out a survey asking nurses how they perceive or rate the responsiveness of individual practitioners. Although this method appears more objective, the organization may attain little or no data depending on how the survey is structured and who the survey targets. Asking nurses to record data on physician response times on a medical/surgical unit would be logistically difficult because nurses are not always near the nursing station when the physician arrives. It may, however, be feasible to have the unit secretary record the physician's arrival time. Systematizing the routine and concurrent collection of this data would be more feasible in an intensive care unit where nurse/patient ratios are 1:2.

Another way to actively collect perception data is to include the call and response times into patients' medical records. If the organization uses an electronic medical record (EMR), data relating to response times would be simply a byproduct of care. Systematizing the active collection of such data on a measurable data element (e.g., response times) through the EMR turns what would otherwise be considered perception data into quantitative clinical data because it removes the subjective element (e.g., whether others perceive that a physician responds to call on time).

Although perception data is typically used to evaluate behaviors, if there is a well-defined behavior that the hospital can measure more objectively, such as hand-washing techniques, perception data are not necessary.

Who Should Share Perceptions of Practitioners?

Medical staffs should collect perception data from individuals who can validly evaluate the performance area being measured without bias. Typically, such individuals include the following:

- Peers

- Coworkers

- Supervisors

- Patients and their families

- Referring practitioners or practitioners that receive referrals

Two conditions are necessary to obtain valid perception data:

- The perceiver must be in a position to reasonably observe performance

- The perceiver must have the appropriate knowledge or understanding to evaluate the performance

Who to ask might seem obvious, but medical staffs have historically accepted practitioner evaluations from peers or leaders who may not have monitored the practitioners' performance, or they never sought information from direct observers. For example, many organizations ask for the department chair's evaluation to satisfy the peer reference requirement at reappointment. It is common for the chair of a large internal medicine department to sign a reappointment or privileging recommendation for a practitioner with whom he or she has had little to no interaction. It is also common for a surgery department chair to evaluate a physician's behavior with the clinical staff, yet the chair has never seen the physician in action in the operating room.

Department chairs may simply trust that any issues regarding a physician's performance would have been brought to their attention—"no news is good news"—and assume that everything is fine. However, keep in mind that unless OPPE reports are relevant and assist the medical staff in determining a physician's clinical competence, they are not doing their job. Tap into the nursing unit managers, operating room director, anesthesiologists, or referring physicians, as these individuals are likely able to provide observation-based feedback.

What Are the Appropriate Questions to Ask Perceivers?

A perceiver with the appropriate knowledge or understanding of the issue is critical to a valid evaluation. Asking the appropriate person the appropriate questions will also help physicians accept the data. For example, it would be unfair to the physician to ask a patient or even a nurse to evaluate the physician's technical skills or judgment. Rather, the physician's peers might best evaluate his or her skills and judgment. However, there are many other dimensions of care, aside from surgical or procedural technique, that nonphysicians might evaluate, including the ability to interact with the clinical team, communicate, and comply with organizational policies, such as performing a timeout prior to a procedure or performing a debriefing following a procedure.

For example, it is appropriate to ask a patient whether the physician is a good communicator, for two reasons. First, evaluating whether another person communicates well does not require technical knowledge because the key consideration is whether the message was understood. Second, the patient has less bias than a clinical staff member because the patient does not necessarily know medical terms and therefore can judge whether the communication was clear.

How Should Perception Data Be Collected?

There are two predominant types of perception data: passive and active. Passive perception data are data that are not specifically solicited. Examples of passive data are incident reports, complaints, and compliments. These data are typically based on individual events. They are passive because the data request is not initiated by the group that will use the data. Active perception data are obtained when the user of the data solicits the information from an individual or a group. Examples of active data are evaluation forms, focus groups, surveys, forms, and survey interviews. Usually the solicitor will structure this data using a series of questions or ratings.

Active perception data have several advantages over passive methods, including the following:

- Specific questions can be asked to evaluate specific expectations.

- Data can be aggregated from many individuals to minimize the potential for personal bias of a single individual.

- Data can be aggregated to allow for interpretation within a comparative group rather than an absolute standard. This is particularly important because validating an absolute rating score is much more difficult than validating a comparative score. For example, it is more telling to see how many peer complaints you have in comparison to other practitioners, rather than the absolute or raw volumes on their own.

TIP

The Greeley Company has identified the following tools to collect perception data:

- **Department chair evaluations**: This traditional tool is still a reasonable starting point, especially if an organization expands it to address all of the general competencies and supplements it with other perception data when the chair has not had the chance to observe performance or interact directly with the physician.

- **Rule indicators for incident reports/complaints**: Defining specific rule indicators for perception-based reports allows the medical staff to aggregate the results and set targets for better interpretation.

- **Patient satisfaction surveys with physician-specific questions**: Most patient satisfaction surveys ask the patient specific questions regarding his or her physician's communication skills and demeanor, as well as the amount of time the physician spent with the patient. Many organizations partner with vendors for patient satisfaction evaluations, such as Press Ganey.

- **Student and resident evaluations of attending physicians**: Teaching institutions already have perception data from their trainees on attending physician performance. Although these evaluations are not uniform across all programs and specialties, many include aspects of professionalism and communication.

- **Staff surveys based on Accreditation Council for Graduate Medical Education (ACGME) resident evaluations**: Some medical staffs have begun to take questions from the ACGME resident evaluation's 360-degree survey tool and adapt them to evaluate the attending staff through surveys of the hospital staff.

- **Internal surveys of physicians and staff:** Many organizations have a staff satisfaction survey for hospital employees that may ask general questions regarding the medical staff. An organization could modify these surveys to obtain physician-specific data.

 © 2011 HCPro, Inc.

Figure 5.1 is a sample perception survey for practitioners that you can send to the clinical staff regarding communication and professionalism.

FIGURE 5.1

SAMPLE PROFESSIONALISM ASSESSMENT SURVEY

Please use the following scale to rate professionalism during the most recent experience with your physician.

The doctor	1 = Poor	2 = Fair	3 = Good	4 = Very good	5 = Excellent
Is approachable					
Takes a genuine interest in the patient's health					
Explores patient's needs and concerns					
Listens carefully					
Answers questions from patient and family members					
Communicates clearly and effectively					
Maintains patient's privacy during exams					
Shows compassion and cares					
Shows respect for patient and family members					
Involves patient and family members in decision-making process					
Maintains appropriate behavior with patient and family					
Has good hygiene (washes hands, wears clean clothing)					

Source: The Greeley Company, a division of HCPro, Inc.

How Often Should Perception Data Be Solicited?

It is not always feasible to collect and report perception data on an ongoing basis. How often is "ongoing" review or evaluation? The evolving national standard for OPPE review is between six and nine months. If an organization evaluates a practitioner every six months, it will likely have three to four review cycles to consider at reappointment or renewal of privileges. If the organization evaluates a practitioner every eight months, it will likely have two to three review cycles to consider at reappointment or renewal of privileges.

Although the majority of indicators will appear regularly on every OPPE report, it is not necessary to collect and report on all indicators on every report. Some indicators are not collected regularly enough to be included in every report. Indicators may appear on reports periodically as they are collected and ready for reporting. A few examples follow:

- A summary of patient satisfaction survey results may be reported biannually or annually and would appear on the OPPE report associated with publishing those results

- Employee surveys may be distributed periodically and would appear on the next OPPE cycle

Even some items that are not considered perception data may be periodically reported on OPPE reports. For example, medical malpractice claims history may be queried annually and would be reported in the next OPPE cycle but may not appear on every OPPE report.

The organization could consider having a section of the OPPE report titled "Periodic Indicator Reporting" for these types of items.

How Should Perception Data Be Interpreted?

Similar to other indicators, perception data is best interpreted through thresholds and comparison groups in addition to case level review where necessary. Defining the thresholds and peer or comparison groups (to whom the practitioner's performance is being compared) up front will likely create better buy-in from the physician staff members. For example, if an organization's call response time policy has a rule-based threshold of two occurrences in a 12-month period, meaning that if a physician does not respond to a call in a timely manner once in one year, the medical staff still considers that acceptable behavior. If the physician fails to respond twice, the medical staff may send an educational letter to the practitioner. A third occurrence in a 12-month period may trigger a focused professional practice evaluation.

As with all physician performance indicators, we need to start with the question, "Why are you different?" as opposed to jumping to the conclusion that there is a true performance issue. The OPPE task force should look at most perception data in comparison to other data, so this question is a valid way to begin to understand the data.

Perception data can also be correlational, which can assist in validating perceived problems. For example, if a practitioner has substandard scores on a patient satisfaction survey and has had staff complaints or incident reports, then there appears to be some cross-validation that a problem may exist. Finally, because the use of perception data is new territory for most physicians, it is critical to create up-front physician engagement for the collection and use of the data.

Establishing Thresholds and Benchmarks to Interpret Performance

The ultimate purpose of OPPE is to provide systematic and timely feedback to practitioners on their performance in competency areas the medical staff deems important. The indicators of the key competencies require clear guidelines on how both the medical staff peer review committee and individual practitioners will use and interpret the data. The first step in giving practitioners feedback is creating thresholds and benchmarks.

The absence of agreed upon thresholds and benchmarks against which performance data is compared invites reviewers (members of the medical staff peer review committee or other committees that evaluate OPPE reports) to apply subjective measures of performance to each practitioner. This means that objective data, which the organization has expended time and resources to collect, undergo a subjective review. Subjectivity results in variability in how the data are interpreted and applied, which adversely affects the credibility of the entire program.

A lack of clearly defined thresholds to compare performance against may lead to inconsistent or unequal evaluation of practitioners and expose the organization to legal challenges.

© 2011 HCPro, Inc.   **85**

Setting appropriate thresholds for the indicator type helps the medical staff set attainable goals and recognize normal performance variation. It also improves inter-rater reliability, meaning that as departments change chairs, practitioners should know that their performance data will continue to be evaluated consistently.

Thresholds help reviewers frame their conversations with privilege holders around the question, "Why are you different?" rather than "Why is your performance bad?" They highlight variations in performance, but the root causes of the variations must still be identified. It is possible that the variation is a result of an expected response, systems issue, data integrity issue, or nonclinical process problem (also known as *common cause variation*). Because there are many possible causes for variations, view thresholds as a call to attention, rather than a call to action. Framing thresholds in this manner will help alleviate practitioners' concerns regarding data misuse.

It may be helpful to think of the OPPE program as a screening process. Just because data collected on a practitioner exceed a given threshold does not mean that there is a performance problem. It merely flags the result and indicates that the organization should take a closer look at the reasons why the results for that practitioner are different from others.

Physician leaders are ultimately responsible for recommending or selecting thresholds based on the recommendations from the OPPE task force. Because the indicator and threshold selection are practitioner-led tasks, the OPPE program will have more credibility amongst the medical staff. Using practitioner-selected indicators and thresholds also assists in meeting Joint Commission Standard MS.08.01.03 that requires the medical staff organization to select or adopt performance measures. In addition, the organization is required to identify triggers for focused professional practice evaluation (FPPE). Many of these may arise from OPPE reports.

Now that we understand why setting thresholds is important, it is time to delve into the specifics. This chapter focuses on the following topics:

- The types of thresholds: relative action (excellent and acceptable thresholds), fixed-action (a single, nonnegotiable threshold), and standard deviation

- Selecting thresholds based on the type of indicators (review, rule, rate)

- Using thresholds to interpret variation

- Resources for establishing appropriate thresholds

- What if thresholds are not readily available?

- Thresholds versus comparisons

- Who should select thresholds and benchmarks?

- Supporting continuous improvement

Types of Thresholds

There are three types of thresholds: relative-action, fixed-action, and standard deviation.

Relative-action thresholds

Setting a low and a high threshold for certain indicators allows the medical staff to hone in on acceptable and excellent performance (similar to how medical staffs handle core measures or pay-for-performance initiatives where an acceptable range is noted). Relative-action thresholds are best suited for indicators tailored for performance improvement as they allow

 © 2011 HCPro, Inc.

for average performance and recognize above-standard performance. When possible, it is always better to have two thresholds rather than one. Doing so drives practitioners toward a higher standard of care and the best possible benchmark. The "acceptable" threshold provides an initial guideline for practitioners who are adjusting to performance evaluations, hopefully appeasing any fears about a new process. The "excellent" performance threshold may also appeal to the competitive nature of practitioners. See Figure 6.1 for a graph describing how relative action thresholds drive performance improvement.

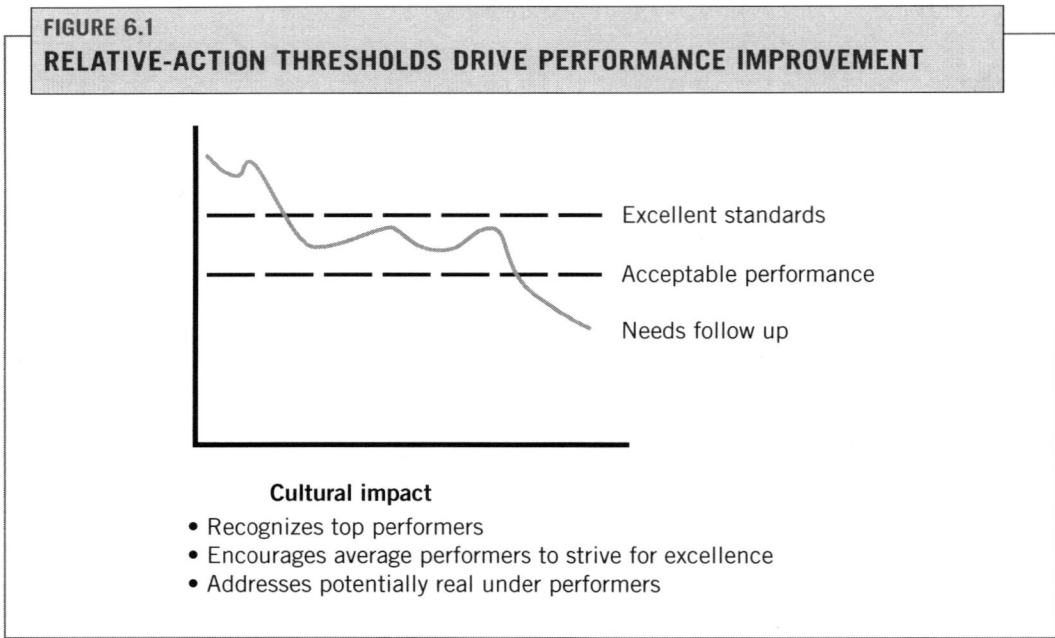

FIGURE 6.1
RELATIVE-ACTION THRESHOLDS DRIVE PERFORMANCE IMPROVEMENT

Excellent standards

Acceptable performance

Needs follow up

Cultural impact
- Recognizes top performers
- Encourages average performers to strive for excellence
- Addresses potentially real under performers

Fixed-action thresholds

Setting a single, nonnegotiable threshold sets the standard for "acceptable" performance. Falling outside of the single threshold helps identify practitioners who fall below adequate standards of care. Once this happens, the medical staff peer review committee should consider an intervention, possibly via FPPE. The OPPE task force often selects fixed-action thresholds when zero defects are the objective of a measure that has an immediate effect on patient safety. See Figure 6.2 for a graph describing how fixed-action thresholds focus on underperformance.

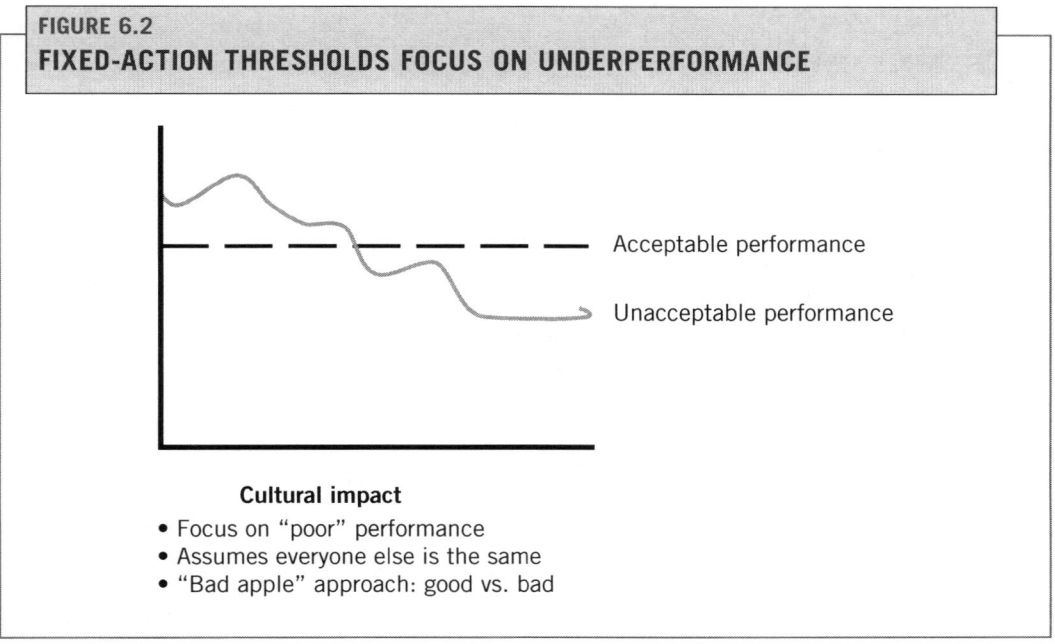

FIGURE 6.2
FIXED-ACTION THRESHOLDS FOCUS ON UNDERPERFORMANCE

Acceptable performance

Unacceptable performance

Cultural impact
- Focus on "poor" performance
- Assumes everyone else is the same
- "Bad apple" approach: good vs. bad

Standard deviation thresholds

Standard deviation is a commonly used measurement of variability. It is a more sophisti-cated threshold and requires a basic understanding of statistics. Demonstrating perfor-mance variation from the mean (average or expected value) gives context to an indicator by comparing a practitioner's performance to that of his or her peers. A low standard deviation signifies that the overall results (or data points) for an indicator are close to the mean. A high standard deviation signifies that the results extend over a wide range of values. In general, we do not expect a large variation in patient care outcomes from practi-tioner to practitioner. For patient care indicators, there's an expectation to see a certain level of standardization and to see results spread closer to the mean. Hence, consider using lower standard deviations as thresholds, such as one-half or one standard deviation away from the mean, in order to capture true performance issues.

Consider using standard deviation as a threshold when acceptable and when excellent performance thresholds are either reliant on or relative to peers' performance. Determine the most appropriate peer comparison group for the indicator. The group may include practitioners from the same specialty or hospitals, or the comparison might focus on specific diagnosis or procedures. Also consider the statistical significance of the comparison group (i.e., volumes) to ensure that comparisons are made against a valid sample size.

Adjusting Data for Patient Severity/Acuity and Case Complexity

When possible, internal benchmarks should take into account the severity (acuity) and complexity of the patient population to allow for an apples-to-apples comparison. One of the common methodologies for severity adjustment is the 3M™ All Patients Refined Diagnosis-Related Groups (APR DRG). This software uses information collected from the coding and billing process to adjust patient data for severity of illness ("How sick is the patient?") and risk of mortality ("How likely is it the patient will die?") and classifies it.

However, such software may be too costly and beyond the reach of many organizations. If this is the case, you may elect to include easily available information, such as the case-mix index (CMI) in the OPPE reports. CMI is derived from diagnosis-related groups (DRG), which are necessary for inpatient billing purposes and is the average weight of complexity for the hospital's Medicare volume. It carries significant financial implications. The assumption is that the higher the CMI, the higher the acuity and complexity of the patient care, as well as the cost of care. Although this may not always be the case, it is often directionally accurate. Thus, CMI is not used to precisely adjust risk but it does provide a rough rating of the severity of illness as it relates to the intensity of resources required to care for a patient.

In addition to severity adjustment and CMI, narrow the definition of some indicators by excluding specific populations known to influence the results. For example, if a cesarean section (C-section) rate is an indicator selected by obstetricians, consider eliminating populations under the age of 16 or over the age of 35 where a C-section is more likely to occur. This practice is similar to the measure adopted by the Agency for Healthcare Research and Quality (AHRQ) for limiting the measurement of mortality to low-mortality DRGs. Another example is if an organization monitors anesthesiologists' performances relative to thermoregulation, it may exclude trauma patients admitted from the field or procedures where hypothermia is a specific objective. This approach limits the influence of factors unrelated to practitioner performance on the measure and assists in improving specificity.

When using this approach, the OPPE task force should look for adverse information where it does not expect to find it, and minimize the effect that high-risk patients have on the outcomes. Some patients, no matter what a practitioner does, will have negative outcomes due to the presence of comorbid conditions, etc. These patients should be considered, but their outcomes should not weigh more heavily in the OPPE report than lower risk patients.

The APR DRG and CMI apply to inpatient cases. As of 2011, there is no nationally recognized severity adjustment methodology for physicians' hospital based outpatient cases (such as day surgery, ED or observation patients). Include other parameters in the OPPE report to supplement or to replace the CMI and provide the reviewer with a preliminary indication of why a particular practitioner's results are different from his or her peers. These include the average patient age, source of admission, length of stay, or other characteristics that might have implications to patient acuity or the likelihood of comorbid conditions.

TIP

For more information on the APR DRG visit: *http://solutions.3m.com/wps/portal/3M/en_US/3M_ Health_Information_Systems/HIS/Products/APRDRG_Software/.*
For more information on CMI visit: *http://www.cms.gov/.*

If an indicator definition is so broad that it includes large populations of high-risk patients, the organization may find it difficult to use the indicator productively. The goal is to build specifications for the indicator that isolate, to the extent possible, the direct influence of practitioner behavior on the outcome.

Who Should Select Thresholds and Benchmarks?

The stakeholders who selected the indicators for the OPPE program should also select the thresholds. Selecting thresholds does not have to happen at the same time as the indicator

 © 2011 HCPro, Inc.   THE COMPLETE GUIDE TO OPPE

selection process. Separating the two tasks allows the OPPE task force to perform initial research on what thresholds are available for the indicators selected, rather than spending time researching available thresholds for the entire list of indicators.

If external or internal benchmarks are not available, the OPPE task force should attempt to create thresholds from historical data and present these recommendations to the practitioner leaders who selected the indicators. Then present the recommendations to medical staff leaders and the medical executive committee (MEC) for approval. With this accountability structure in place, physician leaders will have the confidence to uphold OPPE standards. It will also give the medical staff leadership greater leverage in explaining expectations to practitioners, particularly if practitioners express concern about certain indicators or thresholds. Physician leaders should also explain to the medical staff that the thresholds are not set in stone and will be reviewed and revised regularly (as defined by the OPPE policy) to ensure that they reflect current standards, provide value, and measure areas of interest.

Identifying Resources for Appropriate Thresholds

Locating reliable thresholds is often challenging. Consider both internal and external resources for developing thresholds.

Existing hospital/department benchmarks

The first source for thresholds should come from existing resources if the OPPE task force determines that they provide value. Internal benchmarks have already been vetted and approved by various stakeholders within the organization, reducing the amount of pushback from practitioners. Practitioners may consider being compared to peers a greater source of motivation than external benchmarks because internal benchmarks are more relevant to their everyday practices. Internal benchmarks can often take into account hospital-specific factors, including the type of hospital, such as critical access, teaching, or trauma center. They can also adjust for situational conditions, such as location, socioeconomic aspects (uninsured population, access to healthcare, language barriers, and income levels), and other circumstances that make these benchmarks more valuable to practitioners than some external measures.

With that said, hospitals have more in common than they think. In fact, arguments asserting that a particular hospital is unique and therefore should be exempted from a given standard of care or have a lower standard of performance are not acceptable from the perspective of the community that the hospital serves.

National and specialty organizations

Many organizations submit data to normative databases, which provide broad benchmark comparisons. Examples include federal and state electronic claims databases and specialty society-specific databases. If an organization already expends resources reporting to these databases, it should leverage the data reported by using the results internally on OPPE reports.

Specialty societies often have proprietary adjustment methodologies specific to the types of cases typically seen by those specialty practitioners, which may provide the most accurate benchmarks. Many of these organizations are mentioned in Chapter 3 as external resources for indicators and include the American College of Cardiology and the Society for Thoracic Surgery.

Using benchmarks from prominent societies often reduces the potential for practitioners to argue that the organization's OPPE reports are unreliable or invalid. However, prior to using national and industry standards, identify where the hospital falls in comparison to the benchmarks. If the hospital's performance is low, it may set an unrealistically high initial threshold; if the hospital's performance is high, the task force may consider setting even higher thresholds than the benchmarks.

Research and technology firms

Hospitals often have relationships with healthcare research firms and technology vendors for various purposes across the hospital. Find out what memberships and contracts the hospital has with such organizations and solicit information from them. For example, the Advisory Board Company has several levels of membership that give hospitals access to research, which often feature best practice benchmarks.

Similarly, healthcare technology vendors often track huge amounts of data from hospitals across the country and may be able to provide benchmarks for common indicators. For example, core measure vendors, such as Premier, Core Option, and ACS-MIDAS+, may have benchmarks from various hospitals. Crimson Continuum of Care, a practitioner performance management tool, provides proprietary benchmarks for various quality indicators from cohorts of member hospitals.

Academic journals and literature reviews

Research studies published in academic sources provide helpful benchmarks for thresholds. Because academic literature is often peer reviewed for validity and published in recognized journals, practitioners are less likely to argue against the benchmarks. However, performing extensive literature reviews requires resources.

Due to the constantly changing academic findings, the OPPE task force needs to continually evaluate the literature to stay up to date. It will also be important to ensure that the calculation methodology used for the indicator is the same as the calculation used in the literature from which the threshold is attained. Organizations that use published indicators often conduct periodic environmental surveillance or engage an industry expert or consultant to assess their conformance to contemporary industry standards and best practices.

Academic healthcare journals include *The Journal of the American Medical Association* (*JAMA*), *The Archives of Surgery*, the *New England Journal of Medicine*, and other peer-reviewed subspecialty journals and publications.

What if published thresholds are not readily available?

If thresholds are simply not available for an indicator in the OPPE program, create an internal benchmark using historical data or arrive at a threshold based on peer consensus. Use data collected from manual formats (e.g., in spreadsheets and databases) or in internal data systems that automatically collect performance data. Review the historical data for an indicator and trend it to determine thresholds. Looking at the spread of the data in a graphical format may help the OPPE task force visualize potential thresholds that are most relevant to that indicator. Set reasonable thresholds based on the analysis of historical data as a starting point and use experience to validate and update them as appropriate.

For example, if an internal threshold is set too low and a majority of the practitioners exceed the threshold, further analysis should show that either the practice was acceptable and the threshold needs adjustment, or there is a broader issue that requires a global solution. Alternatively, if an internal threshold is set too high and no one can meet it, either the indicator is unnecessary or the threshold needs to be revised. The risk of using historical data from the organization is that the thresholds may reinforce a substandard level of performance that should be challenged or changed. Avoid subjectivity by documenting the methodology and validating it by testing for external factors that may influence the results.

Selecting Thresholds Based on Indicator Types

Consider the indictor type when selecting thresholds. Consider the following thresholds for the different indicators.

Review indicator

Review indicators flag serious or complex events for further analysis, and by definition, do not always require thresholds. Every outlying case requires a case/chart review. However, some hospitals allow some leeway and apply thresholds that are often at very low target levels. This can be accomplished by assigning a low nominal occurrence threshold. For example, occurrence X triggers a review if it occurs more than three times in a set time frame.

Practitioners often worry that a case review can become subjective and inconsistent. Standardizing the process and the tools that support the process addresses these concerns and improves inter-rater reliability. Figure 6.3 provides a listing of items that organizations may include on a case review analysis questionnaire to guide the evaluation of review indicator outliers.

© 2011 HCPro, Inc.

FIGURE 6.3

SAMPLE CASE REVIEW ANALYSIS QUESTIONS

Outcome

- No adverse outcome

- Minor adverse outcome (complete recovery expected)

- Major adverse outcome (complete recovery not expected)

- Catastrophic adverse outcome (e.g., death)

Effect on patient care

- Care not affected

- Increased monitoring or observation (e.g., vital sign checks)

- Additional treatment or intervention (e.g., IV fluids)

- Life-sustaining treatment or intervention (e.g., intubation or CPR)

Issue identification

- No issues with physician care

- Issue with physician diagnosis

- Issue with physician clinical judgment or decision-making

- Issue with physician technique or skills

- Issue with physician communication or responsiveness

- Issue with physician diagnostic or treatment planning

> ### FIGURE 6.3
> ## SAMPLE CASE REVIEW ANALYSIS QUESTIONS (CONT.)
>
> - Issue with physician follow-up or follow-through
>
> - Issue with physician policy compliance
>
> - Issue with physician supervision (house physician or allied health professional)
>
> - Other physician issues
>
> **Overall physician care**
>
> - Appropriate
>
> - Controversial
>
> - Inappropriate
>
> **Physician documentation**
>
> - No issue with physician documentation
>
> - Documentation does not substantiate clinical course and treatment
>
> - Documentation not timely to communicate with other caregivers
>
> - Documentation unreadable
>
> - Other physician documentation
>
> *Source: Adapted from The Greeley Company, a division of HCPro, Inc.*

 © 2011 HCPro, Inc.

The aforementioned approach provides a methodology for case reviews that reviewers can consistently apply. Additionally, the rating parameters can be imbedded directly into the tool used to assess a practitioner's OPPE results. After the review is complete, the organization will make a summary determination regarding the outcome of the entire review. To accomplish this, the organization can implement a scoring structure for case review. Many organizations use the following scores to record the outcome of a case review:

- Score 1: No concerns identified. Standard of care met.

- Score 2: Variation from expected standard of care did not originate from the physician. Case referred to applicable operations manager.

- Score 3: Variation from expected standard of care attributed to physician action/inaction. No adverse patient impact resulted.

- Score 4: Variation from expected standard of care attributed to physician action/inaction. Adverse patient impact resulted.

If a case receives a summary score of 3 or 4, it indicates that the reviewer(s) identified performance concerns for that practitioner. However, most organizations make the mistake of focusing only on adverse scores. Remember that scores indicating that a practitioner met the standard of care are positive peer review results. For example, seven of a practitioner's cases undergo a review over the course of a year (due to referrals for review, core measure activity, OPPE triggers, etc.), and the outcome of the reviews resulted in a score of 1 or 2. The case scores should be included in the OPPE report because they affirm clinical competence and represent a positive peer review result. In addition, using a scoring system enables medical staff to leverage the work effort expended on the OPPE program and increases the benefits realized from performance review. If a review indicator reveals more outlying cases than expected and the OPPE task force determines that a few outliers are acceptable, convert the review indicator to a rule indicator.

Rule indicator

Both relative-action and fixed-action thresholds can be used with rule indicators. Although relative-action thresholds are ideal because they facilitate acceptable and excellent quality standards, fixed-action thresholds are best used when standards are static or required. If you use a fixed-action threshold, consider setting it further from the true nonnegotiable limit. Doing so provides for a warning period and opportunity to coach practitioners who struggle to meet the standard before taking more serious actions. Because rule indicators are influenced by overall patient volumes, which vary among hospitals, external benchmarks are not available.

Rate indicator

Use relative-action thresholds when possible with rate indicators to indicate acceptable and excellent performance. Relative-action thresholds often work well when best practice standards shift as hospitals improve patient care over time or when the organization is trying to raise the performance level of an entire group. For example, practitioners may achieve an acceptable patient satisfaction score of 90% and excellent patient satisfaction scores above 95%; however, with improvements over time, these thresholds may be revised such that an acceptable patient satisfaction score is 92% and an excellent score is 97%.

The threshold formats should match the indicator result formats. For example, if readmission rates are represented as percentages, the thresholds should also be defined as percentages rather than a percentile ranking, which may also be available for this indicator.

Once thresholds are selected, track them in the data collection work plan, which is available in the downloadable materials.

Using Thresholds to Interpret Variation

When interpreting data, remember that exceeding a threshold does not automatically mean that corrective action is necessary. It simply triggers the question, "Why is your performance different?" There are three options when it comes to interpreting aggregate data (rule and rate indicators):

1. **Use thresholds to interpret overall performance.** Consider the volume of cases that results in outlier performance. For example, if a practitioner is flagged for readmission rates, how high are the overall case volumes? If the practitioner had five cases, it may indicate that the variation is likely statistically insignificant. However, if the volumes are high and the number of readmissions is high, it may call for further review.

2. **Review a sample of cases.** In instances like the readmission example where a practitioner has high volumes, the reviewer may want to review a sample of the practitioner's cases to identify the root cause of the readmissions. Of course, you cannot do this with every practitioner, but when there is a performance concern, particularly with a common trending pattern over time, a chart review is a helpful tool.

3. **Trend analysis.** Trend analysis helps identify variation in performance over time, particularly with high-volume indicators. For example, a trend analysis will show if there is a spike in a practitioner's length of stay in a particular month; a deeper review of those cases might show that there is an outlier case with drastically high length of stay that is affecting the overall average. If the organization uses trending in its ongoing data analysis, consider designing the capacity to provide a trended data array in your OPPE report.

Thresholds versus comparisons

In addition to thresholds, the OPPE task force may include peer comparison averages for indicators to give practitioners a sense of where they fall in relation to the hospital or specialty average for an indicator. Comparisons should not be used in replacement of thresholds. The peer comparison provides reviewers and practitioners with additional information—not only where the practitioner stands relative to the threshold or benchmark, but also where he or she stands relative to peers.

Differentiating Between Process Deficiencies and Practitioner Performance Issues

When the OPPE task force first selected each performance indicator, it considered whether the indicator would successfully isolate the performance of the individual practitioner from other influences. Once the various evaluators review reports and understand the data, issues may surface, as well as opportunities for operational improvements. It is likely that the organization's current peer review plan includes a pathway for system-based or operational issues to be referred to the appropriate operations manager. Apply the same pathway for operational issues identified in the course of conducting an OPPE.

Consider it a red flag when administrative evaluators or medical staff leaders discover a potentially adverse trend across numerous practitioners. Conduct an evaluation of the OPPE processes and keep in mind that in many of these situations, practitioners have little control over their performance. For example, an inefficient discharge planning process may cause consistently high length of stays. Some activities that contribute to a longer length of stay are within the practitioner's control. However, several are not, such as poor diagnostic test turnaround time or the inability to access services at all times. These types of issues are hard to identify and require discussions among multiple stakeholders, including practitioners, case managers, nurses, and others involved in patient care. Stakeholders may have to closely examine a sampling of patient charts to discover the root causes of the prolonged length of stay.

Identifying common and special cause variation

Understanding common and special cause variation is fundamental to validating the integrity of the data included on the OPPE report and making continuous improvements in practitioner-level reporting.

Common cause variation is variation in the performance evaluation process that is inherent to the process. With any process, many factors may influence the results. When common cause variation is present in a process, it does not make sense to focus on why a particular outcome occurred as it may be impossible to eliminate variation completely. Rather, it is necessary to look at the process overall and determine how to reduce variation not attributed to the practitioners under review.

Special cause variation most obviously appears when practitioner performance results fall outside the thresholds. Usually, special cause variation exists as the result of an identifiable root cause that is not an inherent part of the process—an external factor affecting the process.

Special cause variation may be a sign that a process is basically sound but may be impacted by outside influences. Conversely, common cause variation is a sign that variation exists within the process and fundamental changes to the process are needed to reduce variation and to accurately reflect performance goals.

 © 2011 HCPro, Inc. THE COMPLETE GUIDE TO OPPE

Recognizing special causes and distinguishing them from common causes is critical to effectively interpreting OPPE metrics and making decisions based on trends in data rather than on intuitive reactions. Failing to distinguish between common and special cause variation will likely lead to two types of mistakes in the data review. The first is ascribing a variation or problem to a special cause (e.g., the practitioner's behavior is the source of variation in length of stay) when it may be due to a common cause (e.g., there are access issues to rehabilitation facilities or skilled nursing facilities). The second involves assuming that variation is due to a common cause, rather than a special one (e.g., the practitioner's longer length of stay is due to the fact that the transition plan of care is not well formulated and the practitioner has been remiss in planning for discharge).

The key to process improvement is determining the cause of variation and whether the cause is part of the system. The proper means of addressing process improvement and variation reduction depends on whether common cause, special cause, or both types of variation are involved. Knowing the cause for variation is particularly important when evaluating practitioner performance as it is neither beneficial nor motivating to speak in a punitive manner to practitioners for doing something if the variation is inherent in the process.

Supporting Continuous Improvement

Use thresholds to identify and standardize best practices so that performance constantly improves over time. Revise thresholds to encourage continuous progress and development. Figure 6.4 is a graphical representation of how to use thresholds to raise the bar over time.

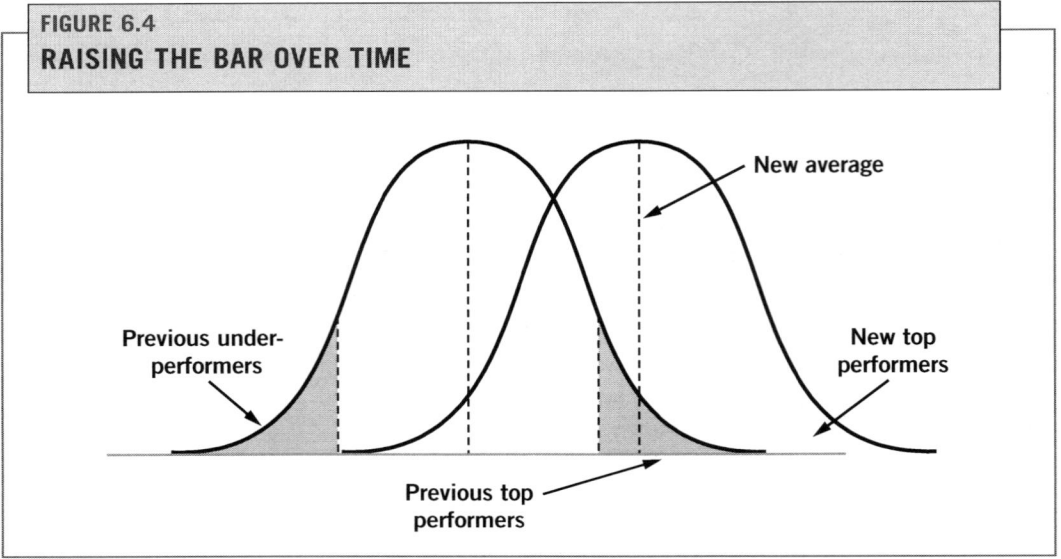

FIGURE 6.4

RAISING THE BAR OVER TIME

New average

Previous under-
performers

New top
performers

Previous top
performers

As discussed earlier in this chapter, it is likely that new and higher benchmarks will evolve over time as the organization strives to raise the performance level of an entire group of practitioners. For example, the organization might initially set a threshold 5% higher than the current level of peer group performance. Once that threshold has been achieved, the organization might decide to push the threshold even higher.

Raising benchmarks is a cause for celebration. Recognize and publicize practitioners' achievements and performance improvements. Celebrating success mitigates the impression that quality improvement programs are punitive and only focus on the bad apples. Additionally, organizations may use evidence that they meet or exceed national thresholds or thresholds espoused by external organizations to market specific programs or in contract negotiations with payers.

Solving the
Attribution Problem

Case attribution is the process of determining which practitioner is primarily responsible for a patient or providing treatment recommendations for a patient. This physician is typically called the "attending" physician. Coders ultimately determine attribution by using the clinical documentation in the medical record as a guide. Because a patient may see multiple practitioners from varying specialties, attribution is an unavoidable pain point that medical staff must proactively address when developing an OPPE process. Attribution is particularly difficult for physicians who have large inpatient volumes comprised of patients who see multiple physicians during their stay. The attribution of hospital-based outpatients to physicians is more straightforward because their patients tend to have shorter hospital stays. This chapter will focus on attribution for inpatients.

Why Is Attribution Difficult?

Although it is possible to list multiple consultants and proceduralists, payers and regulators often require that one practitioner or attending be primarily responsible for the patient. Group-based care, such as hospitalist practices, poses a unique problem because a patient may see several practitioners throughout his or her hospital stay. Consider the following scenario: A patient is admitted through the emergency department (ED) and the ED physician requests an assessment by a specialist. The specialist determines that the patient needs surgery. Complications arise from the surgery and the patient must go to the ICU. Multiple consultants see the patient before he or she is put under the care of a hospitalist team. Finally, a hospitalist discharges the patient. Who should be listed as the attending physician? It is certainly not clear-cut.

Attribution is ultimately determined by the coder who uses clinical documentation in the medical record as a guide to code the case in preparation for billing the payer. Because patients may see several practitioners, coders do not always accurately abstract and code the array of medical professionals who care for a patient. Several institutional factors may contribute to inconsistent attribution processes, including:

- A lack of an organizational attribution policy or procedure that outlines how to select the responsible practitioner/attending, consultants, or other proceduralists who participated in the care of the patient causes variability among coders.

- If a policy does exist, a lack of education amongst coders may result in a subjective attribution process, once again reducing inter-coder reliability. In other words, evaluators may come to different conclusions in their analysis because they lack direction.

- The coder may have difficulty reading the medical record, which may result in attribution of the incorrect physician as the attending physician or omitting a consulting physician.

There is no one solution for the attribution problem. No matter how thorough a process is, the likelihood is that attribution will never be 100% accurate, especially given that accuracy may vary based on individual perspectives. However, take a proactive approach to ensuring that the attribution process is as accurate as possible. Enhance accuracy by creating a comprehensive attribution policy or revising the one your organization already has in place. To create an attribution policy, bring together key stakeholders, including medical staff leaders, coding/medical records personnel, and IT/clinical informatics personnel into a small task force led by the quality/performance improvement department and/or the medical staff services department. It is critical to have physician involvement. The task force's purpose is to:

- Understand the extent of the attribution problem at the organization

- Resolve data integrity issues and minimize errors in data collection

- Develop a consistent and streamlined attribution process that works well for the organization

- Evaluate the new process to assess attribution accuracy rates

Understanding the Extent of the Attribution Problem

Before drafting the attribution policy, the task force needs to understand the extent to which attaining accurate attribution is a problem. Seek answers to the following questions:

- **Does your organization have an attribution policy already in place?** Does it effectively guide the coder in determining the correct attending, consulting, and procedural practitioners? The health information manager, the manager of the coding and medical records department, can typically answer these questions, but he or she may not recognize that a policy is needed or that the existing policy needs revision.

- **Does the medical records department recognize that abstracting for the quality improvement program is part of their responsibility?** Remember that the goal of coding is accurate technical fee billing. The quality improvement professional is now proposing a secondary goal that the department may not recognize as a required work product. The role of the medical records department in the support of the quality improvement program must be established.

- **Do the coders have the training to ensure adherence to these policy?** What medical record leaders believe is the formal attribution process and what the coders do in practice may not be the same. Interview multiple coders to get their perspectives. Keep in mind that some data elements required for OPPE may not be part of the routine record coding process or required to perform technical fee billing. Coders may have to abstract some data for the OPPE program.

- **How accurate are your attribution rates?** The best way to measure the accuracy of current attribution is to audit a sampling of cases. A few subject matter experts (e.g., a clinical quality member, case manager, or medical staff leader) should perform this task. Review the patient charts to determine whether the coder indicated the correct practitioner as the attending. Perspectives may vary but the medical staff, coding department, and other stakeholders, such as the quality department, must discuss these differences and reconcile them as consistently as possible. Consider sampling 5% to 20% of cases across several months to determine accuracy rates for medical and surgical cases separately. Use Figure 7.1 as a template to develop your own audit log.

Alternatively, the organization may elect to design and periodically produce reports that aggregate assignment of practitioners to various case types in an effort to target and drill down on blatant variances or aberrations in abstracting/coding.

FIGURE 7.1

SAMPLE ATTRIBUTION AUDIT LOG

Encounter/patient account number	DRG type	Case attributed to	Accuracy	Details (Reason incorrect/ issues identified)
[Enter patient identifier]	[Medical or surgical DRG]	[Enter admitting physician, discharging physician, provider with the more care time, primary surgeon, or other]	[Enter accurate or inaccurate]	

Solving Data Integrity Issues and Minimizing Data Collection Errors

Incorrect attribution is not just a coding issue. The data coders work with must also be accurate. It is essential to have an accurate roster or inventory of credentialed practitioners. Many organizations refer to these rosters as "doc masters" or "physician master files." Several hospital departments maintain rosters, such as the medical staff services department (MSSD) and billing offices. This can create a data management problem as lists may vary. Because the MSSD is the focal point for onboarding and terminating practitioners, consider designating that department's roster of active, credentialed practitioners as the data source for downstream business applications, including the OPPE process.

Create a policy and procedure for maintaining the roster to ensure it is always up to date. The policy should outline who is responsible for updating the roster, how often that person must update the roster, and how to update other systems affected by changes to the roster.

 © 2011 HCPro, Inc.

> ## TIP
>
> The following are a few common roster inaccuracies that medical staff professionals should watch out for:
>
> - Duplicate names or identification numbers in the roster (e.g., the same provider appears under two IDs or the same ID is used for multiple providers)
>
> - Providers are not tied to the correct specialties (e.g., providers may not be tied to a specialty or may be tied to the wrong specialty)
>
> - Inactive providers on the roster are listed as active
>
> - Inaccurate list of specialties (e.g., specialties aren't listed, are listed twice, or are spelled incorrectly)
>
> - Inconsistent application of specialties or ordering of specialties such as endocrinology as primary for one practitioner and internal medicine as primary and endocrinology listed as secondary
>
> - Inactive practitioners or practitioners in specific categories (such as "Refer and Follow") who do not need to go through the OPPE review process

The IT department can also update or enhance existing systems to help prevent data integrity issues on the roster. For example, consider creating data entry rules, such as:

- Do not allow the use of the same ID more than once in the roster.

- Do not list physicians in certain specialties as the attending. For example, never list emergency department (ED) physicians as attending physicians. Create a list of these specialties and configure IT systems so that they do not allow these practitioners to be selected as the attending.

Hospitals can also use electronic medical records (EMR) and point of service (POS) data collection tools, such as the computerized physician order entry, to reduce attribution problems. EMRs and POS tools provide a direct link between the practitioner making the entry and the patient, procedure, or care order under consideration, thereby eliminating the influence of other participants in data processing.

Developing a Consistent and Streamlined Attribution Process

The medical staff ultimately determines which attribution process an organization implements. Two attribution methods—code based and case time—are described in the following sections.

Code-based attribution

Although some medical staffs create an attribution policy for each specialty, this can be a daunting task. A better option is to establish attribution policies based on case type. Typically, cases can be categorized as either medical, surgical, or OB/GYN. Create a policy outlining the process for each category for how the coder determines who to list as the attending physician and use the diagnosis-related group (DRG) to determine whether a case is medical, surgical, or OB/GYN. This approach makes it easier for coders to consistently choose the correct types of practitioners responsible for the overall management of a patient. For example, if a hospital assigns discharging physicians as attending physicians for medical patients (patients who have a medical DRG), the organization needs to specify whether the discharge physician is the practitioner who completes the discharge order or the discharge summary. Coders also need training on the rules to ensure they assign the correct physician. Additionally, the organization should create rules that will help coders manage expected variances, such as when two practitioners split discharge paperwork.

For surgical cases (patients who have a surgical DRG), the primary surgeon who performs the main procedure is often considered the attending physician because he or she is primarily accountable for the outcomes of care. However, challenges arise when comorbid conditions are exacerbated and postsurgical care is even more complex than the surgery. To overcome this challenge, include caveats in an attribution policy that address such situations. For example, the caveat may state that a case that involves a postsurgical length of stay greater than 10 days would be attributed to the discharging practitioner.

An organization may use DRGs or International Classification of Diseases (ICD-9 or ICD-10) codes to assign OB/GYN patients. These patients are best attributed to the OB/GYN practitioner on the case.

The code-based methodology is a straightforward strategy that makes it easier to train coders and reduce intercoder variability. Although this methodology lessens ambiguity, depending on the organization's culture, the medical staff may not perceive it as accurate enough.

Figure 7.2 is a flow chart outlining the code-based attribution process.

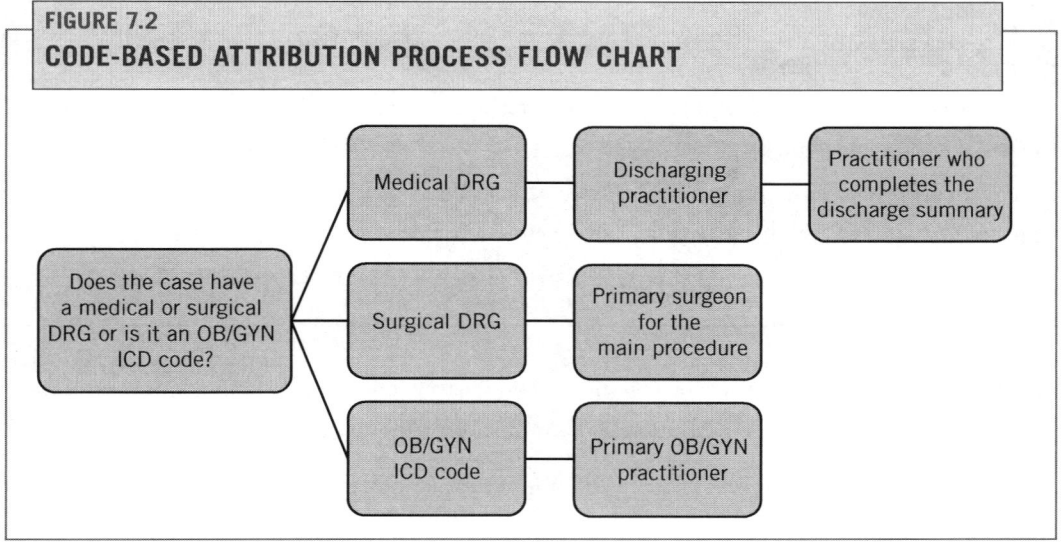

FIGURE 7.2

CODE-BASED ATTRIBUTION PROCESS FLOW CHART

Case-time methodology

Another option is to assign patients to physicians based on the amount of time the practitioner spends caring for the patient. Organizations that use the case-time method assign cases to the specialty or service that provides the most care to a patient. The amount of care is determined by looking at specific metrics, such as progress notes or number of days. Cases are then assigned to the practitioner within that specialty who spent the most time caring for a patient.

© 2011 HCPro, Inc.

> **TIP**
>
> The case-time methodology requires significant staff time to calculate which practitioner spent the most time with the patient and should be listed as the attending. Calculating the time for patients with short stays is often burdensome, so consider adding language to your attribution policy that states that patients who are admitted for less than 48 hours will be attributed to the discharging practitioner, based on the discharge summary or the actual order for discharge.

Although the case-time attribution methodology is a complex process and is time consuming for coders (resulting in possible lower intercoder reliability), it may be more accurate in identifying which practitioner was truly responsible for the patient care outcomes.

Anticipate complexities

No matter whether an organization implements the code-based or the case-time methodology, unforeseen complexities must be accounted for. When possible, determine attribution by outcome or indicator. This can help account for multiple practitioners' involvement in patient care. For example, with the appropriate technical tools it is possible to attribute core measures to specific practitioners (e.g., the admitting physician is assigned core measures specific to admit times).

Practitioners must be allowed to reassign cases on a case-by-case basis. Educate and train them on the attribution methodology and the process for overriding the attribution on a case. This is particularly helpful when a colleague discharges a patient as a professional courtesy.

Weekend discharges can be especially challenging because it is common for the patient to be discharged by a practitioner other than the one who has been treating the patient. The attribution task force should put a policy into place that allows practitioners to reassign cases or to review all weekend discharges on Monday to validate the attribution. Bed assigners and case managers may be good resources to help reassign cases when necessary.

The academic setting can also be challenging because residents typically write orders for tests and medication under the attending physician's name. Two possible solutions are to either have the resident care for patients under his or her own name or to have the resident write orders under a single designated practitioner who is primarily responsible for the resident's learning. Some organizations believe that the resident should enter patient orders under the attending physician because the attending is ultimately responsible for the resident's work and training.

When it comes to group-based care, such as that provided in a hospitalist practice, it makes the most sense to review performance as a group. Although OPPE requires every hospitalist to be evaluated individually, if outlier performance is detected, the medical staff should conduct a more thorough data review at the group level. For example, if an organization has three groups of hospitalists, each group should be evaluated separately and possibly even compared to each other for additional insight.

Evaluating the New Attribution Process to Assess Accuracy Rates

Once the new attribution policy has been implemented, it is important to evaluate its success. Conduct audits identical to the ones you performed prior to developing the new policy so that you can compare accuracy rates before and after implementing the new policy.

As with the overall OPPE policy, it is important that medical staff leadership, for example the medical executive committee, approve the attribution process. Once you create a draft policy, obtain documented authorization or acknowledgement from departments involved in the process, such as patient access, medical records, and possibly IT. Ultimately, the medical executive committee must approve the policy. Once the policy is approved, ensure all stakeholders receive education and training on the new process. Stakeholders may include medical staff practitioners, quality department personnel, medical staff, office staff, and, most importantly, medical records and coding/abstracting staff.

One of the primary reasons for creating a better attribution policy is to enfranchise the medical staff in performance improvement by enhancing data quality. Communicate these reasons for developing a new attribution policy while explaining that 100% accuracy is simply unattainable. Emphasize that the data are used to determine patterns and trends, not to pinpoint blame. Although there is no perfection, the new process is the best possible solution.

Developing Protocols for Low-Volume Practitioners and Advanced Practice Professionals

As the OPPE task force develops the OPPE program, it must address the issues of low-volume practitioners and advanced practice professionals (APP). There are several reasons why there may be insufficient data available for OPPE. A few examples include:

- The practitioner's specialty may be primarily consultative. Although the practitioner is exercising cognitive privileges, patient encounters may not routinely appear on clinical activity reports, which tend to capture procedural activities.

- Abstracting and coding efforts may extend to admitting practitioners or operative physicians of record and not to privileged APPs or consultative activities.

- The organization may not be the primary admitting facility for the practitioner, so the practitioner rarely uses the facility.

The task force must create a process for conducting OPPE when there is insufficient data and the standard OPPE report template or approach cannot be used.

Defining the Low-Volume Practitioner Problem

The Joint Commission requires medical staffs to conduct OPPE on all practitioners with active privileges. Do not confuse medical staff membership with privileges—they are two distinct determinations, each with its own criteria for clinical activity:

1. **Clinical activity requirements related to membership:** The medical staff's governing documents, which define the number of procedures, consultations, patients admitted, or patients referred to the organization to qualify for specific staff categories such as active, associate/affiliate, or honorary status.

2. **Clinical activity requirements related to privileging:** Privilege forms reference clinical activity maintenance requirements for continuation of privileges.

Any practitioner who has been granted clinical privileges for the provision of patient care must undergo OPPE. Medical staff leaders, such as department chairs or clinical service chairs, determine what defines competency for the privileges that a practitioner holds. Evidence of ongoing clinical practice for procedure-based practitioners is determined primarily by clinical outcome data. For example, a gastroenterologist with colonoscopy privileges must complete at least (n) number of colonoscopies during a one-year period as part of the eligibility criteria to obtain or maintain the privilege. Most minimum clinical activity requirements are for a 24-month period, so monitoring maintenance criteria for individual privileges at OPPE intervals is not feasible. However, clinical activity occurring at or near to renewal of privileges may be included as part of the OPPE reports.

Conducting OPPE for low-volume practitioners is difficult because there is not a lot of data on their performance. Medical staff professionals or quality staff often struggle with collecting data from sources when the practitioner only visits the hospital and exercises privileges a few times per year. Regardless of the source of data, the key is to obtain enough information to make an accurate judgment of a practitioner's competence.

Identifying Data Sources and Managing Low-Volume Practitioners

Although gathering data is difficult, there are several options for managing low-volume providers.

External sources

If a physician does not perform the minimum number of procedures required, the medical staff services department may depend on the relationship with other facilities in the area to supplement internal findings with information or data obtained from other facilities where the practitioner holds similar privileges. If local competing facilities do not share individual practitioner outcomes, place the burden of obtaining clinical data to support/supplement OPPE on the practitioner. Some organizations have a statement in the privilege form or in their bylaws stating that it is the practitioner's responsibility to provide clinical data and any other information deemed necessary to make competency decisions, and that failure to supply requested information may affect the practitioner's eligibility for a specific privilege.

Refer-and-follow privileges

Refer-and-follow privileges grant a practitioner the ability to visit with his or her patients, review their medical records, and discuss the cases with attending physicians. This type of privilege is often used when a primary care practitioner routinely refers the care of a patient requiring hospitalization to a hospitalist. Practitioners who have refer-and-follow privileges do not have privileges to write orders or progress notes or to make independent treatment decisions. OPPE is not required for these practitioners as they do not have active privileges and do not provide patient care services at the hospital.

As an alternative to refer-and-follow privileges, medical staffs may chose to grant low-volume practitioners "dependent privileges." Dependent privileges require another practitioner to participate in the care of a low-volume practitioner's patients. For example, an active practitioner may comanage patients with a low-volume practitioner, serve as a mandatory consultant on all cases, or assist the low-volume practitioner during surgical procedures. If the medical staff chooses to grant dependent privileges, it must consider the political ramifications of fee structures, who pays for the assisting physician, reimbursement issues for consulting physicians associated with a dependent low-volume practitioner, and medical malpractice coverage. The organization should place the burden on the applicant to obtain the requisite supervision or comanagement services.

Medical staffs may also grant low-volume practitioners membership but not privileges. Granting practitioners membership without privileges enables them to participate in meetings and, in some cases, vote on medical staff decisions. They also have the ability to network with the entire medical staff, participate in functions, and gain access to continuing medical education or other educational programs.

In many instances, physicians that practice only in the ambulatory setting and do not directly admit patients to the hospital are satisfied with medical staff membership and have no interest in obtaining clinical privileges for inpatient treatment. The medical staff organization may create dependent, refer-and-follow privileges, or another option for practitioners who want to have membership without privileges.

Authoritative references

The objective of OPPE is to evaluate the ongoing performance of clinical privileges using firsthand internal data from the hospital where a practitioner holds those privileges. However, Joint Commission Standard MS.07.01.03 offers an alternative option when there is insufficient internal information. It states that when evaluating an applicant for privileges, the medical staff may use peer recommendations if there are insufficient peer review data available. Best practice is for the querying facility to accept only an "authoritative" reference attesting to a practitioner's competence to perform privileges requested. Authoritative references include a department chair or medical staff leader at a hospital or outpatient center where the privilege holder exercises the scope of privileges requested.

Peer recommendations sometimes cannot be provided because the privilege holder has not exercised the requested privileges at any facility during the previous 24 months. In that event, the practitioner is unable to provide evidence of ongoing clinical competence, and there may be no real basis for continued privileging. When deciding whether there is sufficient information to continue specific privileges, the organization may also evaluate whether the applicant for renewal has sufficient evidence of ongoing clinical activity and competence in advanced privileges. If the applicant meets the criteria for advanced privileges, the organization may determine that he or she also meets the privileging criteria for less complex privileges that require related skills and knowledge.

TIP

Regardless of the method of obtaining data for OPPE for low-volume practitioners, there are a few key points that Joint Commission—accredited hospitals should consider regarding data collection from other facilities and defining policies around low- and no-volume providers. The Joint Commission highlighted these issues in its March 23, 2010 FAQ, which is available at *www.jointcommission.org/standards_ information/jcfaqdetails.aspx?StandardsFAQId= 311&StandardsFAQChapterId=74.*

 © 2011 HCPro, Inc.

Addressing Low-Volume Practitioners in the OPPE Policy

To ensure equity, the OPPE policy should outline specific permissible options for low-volume practitioners. The following are a few examples of processing options that the OPPE task force can stipulate in the policy in the event of insufficient data to produce a report:

- If there is insufficient data for one review period, the department chair may elect to continue monitoring the patient care provided by the practitioner. However, if there are two consecutive periods of insufficient information, the organization might elect to obtain an authoritative external peer reference regarding the performance of similar privileges at the practitioner's primary practice location.

- If a practitioner has less than (n) patient encounters or cases at an organization during a review period, the organization may conduct a case review at the next available opportunity. If the practitioner has not had any clinical activity for the entire 24-month period at the evaluating hospital and the evaluating hospital does not have a specific minimum requirement for patient contacts that must occur during a 24-month period, the organization may obtain an authoritative external peer reference regarding the performance of similar privileges at the practitioner's primary practice location.

- If the practitioner has not had any clinical activity at the organization during the 24-month period and the evaluating organization has a minimum requirement for patient contacts for a practitioner to qualify for renewal of privileges or member-ship, the practitioner may be terminated or may be considered ineligible to apply for privileges.

 © 2011 HCPro, Inc.   THE COMPLETE GUIDE TO OPPE

- In lieu of clinical activity data from another facility, the organization may accept an authoritative peer reference from an organization where the practitioner has similar privileges. The department chair or another medical staff leader who can attest to the clinical competency or provide a privilege recommendation completes the authoritative reference. The organization requesting the information selects the "authoritative source," typically a peer in a position of authority at the alternative facility. The practitioner under review should not select the source. Although the requesting organization does not have sufficient clinical activity to generate or aggregate data, the practitioner may have enough clinical activity at the other facility for case review.

Selecting Indicators for APPs With Supervised Privileges

APPs are practitioners other than licensed physicians who provide direct patient care services in the hospital/medical center under a defined degree of supervision by a physician medical staff member who has been granted clinical privileges. APPs, such as physician assistants, psychologists, and advanced practice registered nurses, are credentialed and privileged through the medical staff and are therefore subject to OPPE.

Obtaining aggregated, trended data for APPs can be difficult. Because the clinical activity of these individuals has not been traditionally abstracted and coded through medical records, data regarding something as basic as clinical activity may not be available from traditional sources. In the past, if an APP was involved in the care of a patient, the outcomes were attributed to the attending physician. However, the demands of data reporting require more accurate attribution. The medical staff should recognize that oversight for clinical privileges exercised by these individuals is just as important as oversight for physicians. Accreditation agencies expect organizations to conduct the same surveillance and peer review for APPs as for physicians.

In circumstances where APPs have been granted the same privileges as physicians, the same indicators can apply. For example, perioperative thermoregulation is just as important when a physician administers general anesthesia as when a certified registered nurse anesthetist (CRNA) administers general anesthesia. If that indicator is applied to physicians with these privileges, it should also apply to CRNAs with the same privileges. There is no reason why the same strategy for data collection could not apply.

If the organization has implemented a field-level electronic medical record (EMR), the OPPE task force may not need outside resources, such as coding staff, to obtain data on APPs. Rather, the medical staff may work with EMR stakeholders to ensure the screen includes fields to capture information regarding advanced practice professionals and feed it into the OPPE report.

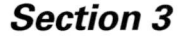

Section 3

Compiling OPPE Reports and Implementing the OPPE Program

Designing Practitioner-Friendly OPPE Reports

As with any reports or written communications, there is always the risk that practitioners will ignore OPPE reports or take only a cursory interest, particularly if the contents are hard to understand. The reality is that practitioners have demanding schedules and do not have time to decipher an encrypted message. The role of the OPPE task force is to mitigate this risk by presenting the data and designing a report in such a way that will engage practitioners' interest and intellectual curiosity. It is not enough to simply have all the data in the report; instead, the data must be turned into information through thoughtful layout and structure.

During the report design and delivery process, keep in mind the following factors that may influence how the medical staff receives OPPE reports:

- Medical staff culture: As with the delivery of any communication, keep in mind the nature, motivations, and predispositions of the audience. What is the hospital's relationship with the medical staff? What is the medical staff's current attitude around performance improvement and practitioner reporting? If there are concerns regarding performance improvement and practitioner reporting, what precautions

© 2011 HCPro, Inc.   **129**

must the OPPE task force take to ensure that medical staff members do not regard OPPE reports as punitive?

- Purpose of OPPE: What message does the medical staff want to deliver? What is the medical staff's end goal when conducting an OPPE? How should the OPPE task force communicate those goals through OPPE reports? How responsive are practitioners to performance improvement? What will appeal to them or stimulate their interest?

The main goal of designing OPPE reports is to turn the data into meaningful information as the success of an OPPE program depends on whether the medical staff hears the message about the organization's goals for practitioners' performances, how those goals are communicated, and whether the goals translate to the practitioners' individual performances. That information must be transformed into actions that result in performance improvement or confirm clinical competence.

The OPPE task force must design the structure and format for OPPE reports. Ideally, the medical staff leaders in the group will take a proactive approach and share their thoughts from a practitioner's perspectives. The OPPE task force must resist temptation to think of delivering reports as a procedural task to simply get the data out to the practitioners. Instead, consider the medical staff culture and the goals for OPPE when considering the following elements of the report:

- Organization of the data to design a meaningful report structure

- Inclusion of key information to report the data

- Interpretation of OPPE reports using thresholds and comparisons

Organizing Data by Competency Framework

Often, hospitals organize reports by disease areas; for example, chronic obstructive pulmonary disease (COPD) care and outcomes will include COPD patient mortalities, complications, readmissions, length of stay, and so on. If the OPPE task force based the OPPE program on the six competency categories recommended by the Accreditation Council for Graduate Medical Education, the indicators in the report should reflect that same structure. In the COPD example, the clinical outcomes would be placed in the patient care category, the resource-related indicators in the systems-based practice category, and the nonclinical indicators in the other appropriate categories. This moves the focus from patient care to the patterns of care within the general competencies, which provides a more robust performance profile.

Separate activity data from performance indicators

Activity-related indicators (e.g., volumes of procedures, admissions, consults) should be separated from performance-related data that fall within the six general competency areas. Separating activity-related indicators from performance-related data will prevent practitioners from assuming that the organization equates volume with performance and is conducting economic credentialing.

Activity or volume criteria may also be included as maintenance criteria for specific privileges, meaning that a practitioner must provide evidence of ongoing clinical practice or perform a certain number of procedures over a specified time period to renew his or her privileges. For example, to be eligible to apply for core privileges in interventional cardiology, an initial applicant must be able to demonstrate performance, reflective of the scope of privileges requested, for at least (n) percutaneous coronary intervention procedures in the past 24 months.

© 2011 HCPro, Inc.

Clinical activity included in OPPE reports typically does not provide case-level information required to meet maintenance criteria for individual privileges. However, including general clinical activity information (i.e., the top five diagnosis-related groups [DRG] or procedures) in the OPPE report can provide context for evaluators, helping them understand the focus of the practitioner's clinical practice and the types of patients to which the indicators/measures were applied.

Many organizations do not provide comprehensive procedure-level information in the OPPE report. Instead of reporting raw clinical activity data, the organization may filter the data to create a snapshot of clinical practice performance. It may be more relevant to include raw data that details procedure-level clinical activity in a separate report at reappointment or renewal of privileges when specific evidence of ongoing clinical practice reflective of the specific privileges requested is of most value.

Using the OPPE report to create a snapshot of clinical practice can be very helpful for evaluators who may not personally know the practitioner under review. When the evaluator does not know the practitioner under review, the OPPE report needs to provide a window through which key information about clinical practice is communicated.

For example, the top five medicine DRGs and the top five surgical DRGs may provide valuable information about where practitioners spend most of their time. This type of snapshot of clinical activity provides context for the other measures/indicators in the OPPE report and provides the user of the report with a backdrop to understand the scope and complexity of a practitioner's clinical practice.

Practitioners with insufficient clinical activity to produce a meaningful OPPE report may be subject to focused professional practice evaluation (FPPE). Insufficient performance information is a common trigger for FPPE.

Specialty-specific reports

There will be some indicators that apply across all specialties, such as patient satisfaction rates or medical records compliance. There may also be some clinical indicators that apply to a particular group of specialties. For example, an indicator that measures how many patients return to the operating room after surgery might apply across all surgical specialties, but not medical specialties. Standardize OPPE reports by specialty and include only the relevant indicators for the physician's specialty. If an indicator is not relevant to a particular practitioner specialty, do not include it in the report. Including nonrelevant indicators in an OPPE report can influence the evaluator and the practitioner's perception of the integrity and relevance of the report.

Including Key Data Elements in the Report

Although keeping reports brief and easy to read is crucial, there are several factors OPPE task forces should consider including in order to give context to the results. Here are a few key elements to consider:

- **Indicator definitions:** If the indicator title is not detailed enough to explain what it measures, consider adding a subtitle or elaborating on the indicator in an appendix. Also, define which indicators are severity adjusted and which ones are not, possibly within the title.

- **Indicator type:** Consider whether defining the indicator type as review, rate, or rule indicator will be important to practitioners. If administrative staff support the

OPPE process and evaluators and individual practitioners are familiar with this language, then consider incorporating the indicator type into the OPPE report. If the indicator type does not add value, or if it confuses evaluators, then exclude it.

- **Indicator results:** Show the calculated value in the results column as opposed to the raw numbers. Do not make the practitioner calculate the results. This concept applies particularly to rate indicators, which use a numerator and denominator. It may be helpful to include the numerator and denominator that created the result in a separate column so that practitioners can understand the data in relation to the volume of activity or sample size. For example, a consultant usage rate of 50% is not meaningful if the numerator is 1 and the denominator is 2.

- **Flexible data time periods within reports:** Not all data become available at the same time. Core measures and severity-adjusted data from external vendors typically have a lag time. Maintain the option to display multiple and different date ranges for different indicators. There is no need to wait until all the data are available for the same period of time to deliver reports. Additionally, if there are not enough data to catch true patterns and issues, consider providing a rolling refresh with a longer time frame so that indicators can be updated at different intervals as data becomes available. Be sure to specify the date range and whether it is a rolling or static comparison.

Helping Evaluators and Practitioners Interpret OPPE Reports

Indicator results need to be presented within the context of the hospital's expectations for performance (using thresholds) and how practitioners are performing in comparison to their peers (using comparative peer data).

Thresholds

Specify the thresholds used for each indicator. Express thresholds in the same format as the indicator results. For example, if the OPPE report expresses readmissions as a percentage, as opposed to a percentile, average, or index, express the threshold as a percentage as well. Otherwise, it is impossible for practitioners to interpret the results.

Rather than using the terms "high" and "low" to describe thresholds, consider using "acceptable" and "excellent," as this language better describes the intent of thresholds (remember, the goal of OPPE is to improve patient care). However, if the medical staff is more familiar with different terms and finds them meaningful, the OPPE task force may continue using them to avoid confusion. Avoid terms such as "fair" because they create confusion over whether a result requires action or follow-up. Terms should clearly indicate when results meet minimum requirements.

Results illustration formats

Visual formats are the most effective way to help practitioners quickly interpret indicator results. It is likely that indicators will be pulled from multiple systems that may have different formats for illustrating results. To create a report that gives practitioners results at a glance, collate the data from the various sources into one standardized report. This will also avoid confusion and frustration with multiple reports, layouts, and definitions.

Whether the OPPE task force chooses color-coded scenarios, graphs, or symbols, use the same format across all indicators and show defined levels of performance, such as "excellent," "acceptable," and "needs follow-up." Avoid colors or symbols associated with negativity as much as possible. The colors the OPPE task force uses will depend on the organization's culture. Some organizations may use green to represent "excellent," yellow to represent "acceptable," and red to represent "needs follow-up." If the medical staff has not seen a color-coded format in other reports, practitioners may perceive a red result as punitive, as red often highlights negative aspects. Instead, consider using white, grey, and blue color highlights, which are less emotionally charged. If practitioners are familiar with the green, yellow, and red concept, it is okay to continue using that color coding to avoid confusion. Although color schemes are arguably the easiest to recognize and interpret, some hospitals use symbols and characters such as a plus sign (+), a zero (0), and a minus sign (−); up, down, or horizontal arrows; one, two, or three stars; and even smiling, neutral, and sad faces (particularly pediatric hospitals, although this may run the risk of being emotionally charged in some organizations).

Whether the task force uses a color scheme, graphs, or symbols to illustrate results, do not assume that practitioners will be able to understand the OPPE report without explanation. Consider using a legend or key at the bottom of each page to define the formats and describe the implications of the results.

Comparative results

Consider comparing an individual practitioner's results to those of other practitioners in his or her specialty or to the hospital average, if such a comparison is appropriate. This helps the practitioner visualize where he or she falls in comparison to peers. Be sure to explain that the comparative results do not define what is "good" or "excellent"—that is the purpose of the thresholds. Comparative results are not typically used as a substitute for thresholds. If necessary, clearly state the difference between thresholds and comparisons in the footer of the report or in a separate document. Comparative results are certainly not critical to understanding performance, but there is no harm in including them.

If, however, an organization has no external or published benchmark or threshold for a particular indicator, it may use comparative data to develop a target or threshold. Using comparative data to develop a threshold is helpful when the organization is trying to increase the level of performance of an entire specialty.

Group-level comparisons

Certain practitioners, such as hospitalists, practice as a group and provide coverage for each other. For such groups, consider including group-level data in the OPPE report in addition to individual data. If the practitioners work as a group, it only makes sense to review their data as a group. Often, hospitals contract with groups and establish group performance expectations, so it is not at all unusual to evaluate group-level performance.

Group-level comparisons can be helpful in environments where specific practitioner attribution is challenging, such as in academic medical centers where faculty supervision of residents can vary daily, attending assignments change based on the date, or an assignment change occurs in the middle of a patient's hospital stay. If an OPPE report unearths a potentially adverse variation in group performance, then the organization may have to isolate the origin of the variance by subjecting the group to FPPE. However, OPPE requires feedback on individual practitioners, so include both group and practitioner-specific data in every report. Consider including an explanation of why both data sets are presented in the report, perhaps as a cover letter.

Figure 9.1 is an example of how to structure an OPPE report.

FIGURE 9.1
SAMPLE OPPE REPORT STRUCTURE

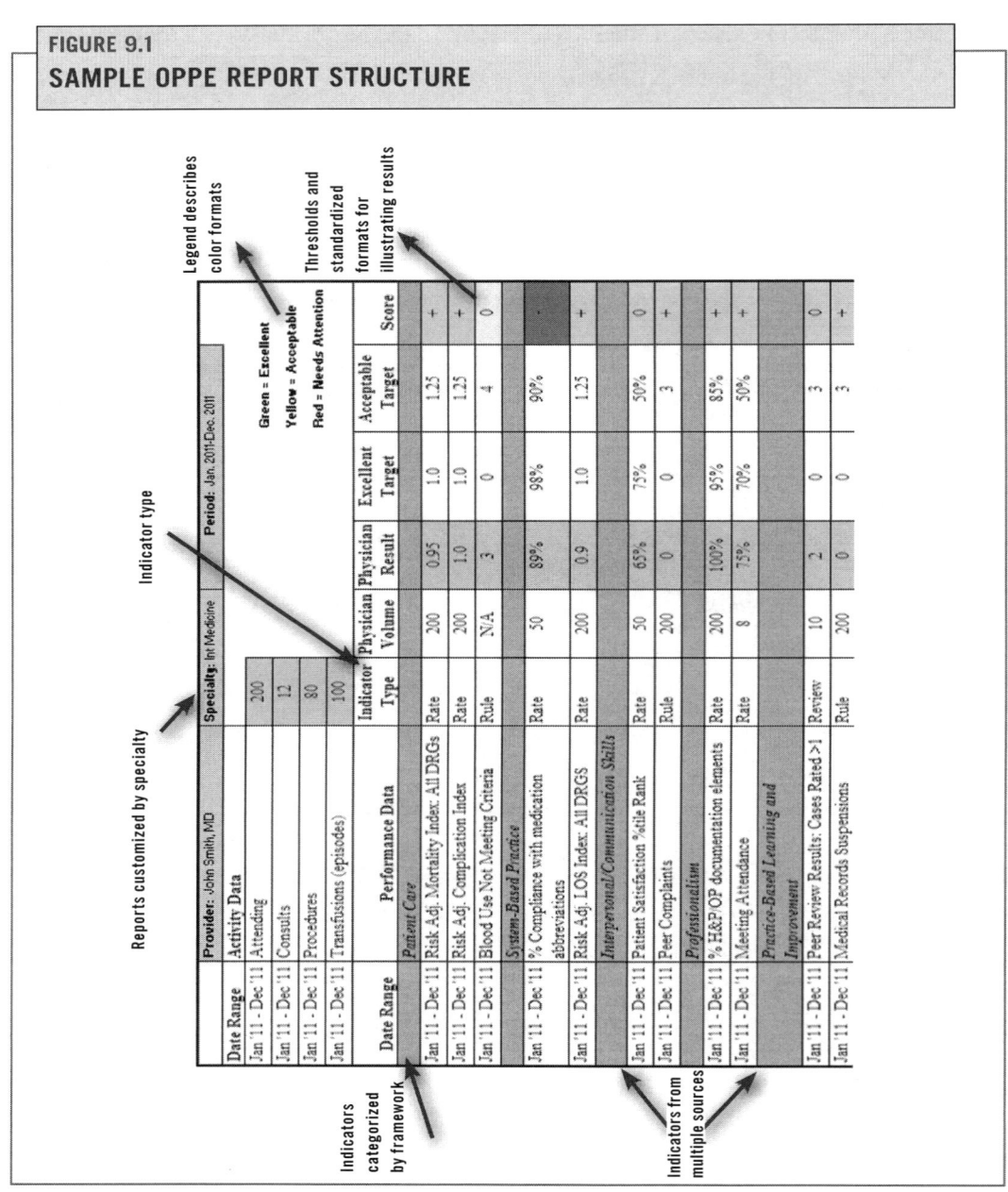

THE COMPLETE GUIDE TO OPPE

Incorporating Supporting Materials to Give Context to OPPE Reports

OPPE reports do not sufficiently establish context for why OPPE is important to the hospital and the medical staff. Without including any context, some practitioners may misunderstand the reason for these reports and fail to see the benefits of a clinical quality improvement program. This may cause unwarranted pushback from practitioners under review. Including supporting materials in OPPE reports helps practitioners understand the context for the reports. Supporting materials include:

- Cover letters

- Explanation of report formats

- Glossary of terms and indicators

- Frequently asked questions (FAQ)

- OPPE policy for additional reference

Cover letters

A cover letter sets the tone for the OPPE reports. Not all practitioners will be familiar with OPPE, no matter how thorough the organization's communication plan. Keep the following tips in mind when drafting cover letters:

- Explain the medical staff's ownership of OPPE, the reason why the reports are being delivered, and why OPPE is important to the hospital and medical staff. Reiterate in the cover letter the key messages on OPPE that the task force developed as part of a communication plan.

- Tailor the cover letter to the type of practitioner, such as attending, consulting, surgeon, group practitioners, low-volume practitioners, or advanced practice professionals. Explain the attribution process and elaborate on unique points applicable to each type of practitioner. For example, consultants often cannot be held solely accountable for patient care outcomes, such as readmissions. Customize the cover letter to explain that the report includes data regarding patients the practitioner consulted on but it is recognized that the responsibility spans across multiple caregivers.

- Include a standard caveat regarding the significance (or lack thereof) of outlier status of indicators if the practitioner's volumes are low. For example, if a practitioner's severity-adjusted complication rates fall outside the set thresholds, but the patient volumes are very low, there is likely little need for concern. Mention that if there are true concerns, the OPPE task force will notify the practitioner. Doing so will help alleviate practitioners' concerns about the repercussions of the results.

- Highlight the final status of the OPPE process. Customize the text to convey whether the individual passes through the OPPE process or whether he or she needs a more in-depth review that might lead to focused professional practice evaluation (FPPE). Explain next steps associated with each status. Highlight or bold these final findings to call attention to them.

- Provide contact information for individuals who can answer any questions practitioners may have—typically a RN in the quality/performance improvement (PI) department or medical staff services department. It is imperative that these individuals are prepared to address common concerns regarding the indicator selection process, attribution, thresholds, possible outlier status, and others.

It is not necessary to create individual cover letters for each practitioner. Instead, create templates for each type of practitioner (attending, consulting, surgeons, group practitioners, low-volume practitioners, or allied health professionals) and the result of OPPE (seamless pass through or FPPE).

Explanation of report formats

Include a brief document with the report that describes the purpose of each field or column and an explanation of how to interpret color or symbol schemes. Another option is to include this information as a legend at the bottom of the report. If the medical staff uses a Web-based or electronic OPPE report, consider including a feature that allows the reader to see definitions or explanations by hovering the cursor/arrow over a column or value.

Glossary of terms and indicators

A glossary of terms and indicators provides practitioners with greater detail on how indicators and thresholds fit into the competency framework. It can also include a list of data sources and thresholds and the calculation methodology. However, only include this additional information if the medical staff thinks it is important. Otherwise it will just be clutter. If there are known limitations in the data or data sources, the OPPE task force may consider disclosing them in the spirit of transparency. However, the medical staff may decide that this information is best explained on a case-by-case basis. This document can be a practitioner-friendly version of your Data Collection Work Plan.

FAQs

Include a document in the OPPE report packet that answers FAQs. Information in the FAQ and cover letter may overlap. Avoid repetition by including the most pertinent points in the cover letter and put the rest in the FAQ. FAQs are particularly helpful when reports are delivered for the first time. Figure 9.2 is a sample FAQ with common questions and suggestions for drafting responses.

 © 2011 HCPro, Inc.

FIGURE 9.2

SAMPLE OPPE FAQ FOR PRACTITIONERS

Why does the medical staff distribute OPPE reports?	Answer this question by focusing on the hospital's goals and expectations for practitioner's performance. Touch on the reasons why understanding practitioner performance is important in today's healthcare environment. Tie this back to key messages in your communication plan.
What are regulatory and accrediting agencies' expectations regarding practitioner competency? How do OPPE reports and this process meet those requirements?	Explain that ongoing monitoring of practitioner competence is an expectation of both accrediting bodies and the Centers for Medicare & Medicaid Services (CMS).
What aspects of competency does the report cover?	Explain the OPPE process, the competency framework used, and how data is gathered and validated.
How are indicators and thresholds selected?	Explain the OPPE practitioner-led initiative and describe the role of medical staff leaders in developing the OPPE program by selecting indicators and thresholds. Also explain practitioners' roles in pilot testing reports. Give details about the participants of the OPPE task force and their roles and responsibilities. State that indicators and thresholds are not set in stone and that OPPE is an evolving process as the organization learns from past experiences.
How is OPPE linked to recredentialing?	Not all OPPE data will be used for reappointment; be clear about which indicators will be used for reappointment decisions.
Where are OPPE data maintained?	The answer to this question will vary by hospital based on the indicators selected and the technology used.

 © 2011 HCPro, Inc. THE COMPLETE GUIDE TO OPPE

FIGURE 9.2
SAMPLE OPPE FAQ FOR PRACTITIONERS (CONT.)

Who will receive the data?	Data are provided to all privileged practitioners. Clearly state that the data are protected under peer review (as appropriate under specific state statutes) and patient safety work plan standards.
Who will have access to the data?	Typically hospitals allow only the individual practitioners and the appropriate medical staff leaders to have access to the data. Be clear about who receives OPPE reports at your hospital and who can review them.
How often will OPPE reports be distributed?	Explain that accrediting bodies do not specify how often medical staffs must conduct OPPE and that the schedule for review conforms with the guidelines provided. Many hospitals distribute OPPE reports every six to nine months.
How should practitioners interpret OPPE reports?	Explain thresholds and how they differ from comparisons. OPPE is only a starting point to performance evaluation, and outlier status does not automatically indicate a problem. In addition to practitioner performance concerns, outlier status could also result from coding/documentation issues and organizational process problems. Additionally, there will always be data limitations that are unavoidable, which is why if there are true concerns, the practitioner will be notified.
What is focused professional practice evaluation (FPPE)?	Explain the circumstances under which OPPE leads to FPPE at your organization
How will the medical staff improve OPPE reports over time?	Explain that the long-term role of the OPPE task force is to ensure that the reports are fine-tuned over time. Some indicators will be retired as performance improves and new indicators will be added; thresholds will be polished; and data limitations will be mitigated.

 © 2011 HCPro, Inc.

Modify the list of FAQs to include any additional questions that arise after practitioners receive the report. Consider including the FAQs in an orientation packet for new practitioners. If there is a website for the medical staff, consider posting the FAQs there as well so that practitioners can refer to them as needed.

Pilot Testing OPPE Reports With Practitioners

The OPPE task force should request formal and structured feedback from the practitioners who are subject to OPPE. Garnering feedback is an effective way to fine-tune the structure, layout, and contents of OPPE reports.

What should be tested?

The OPPE task force should consider what specific aspects of the OPPE reports to test and receive feedback on. Areas that may require feedback include:

- The acceptability of the indicators and thresholds

- The accuracy of the initial data set

- Whether the format is easy to understand

- The effectiveness of the cover letter, keys, legends, and other supporting material

- The mechanism for distribution

To provide adequate feedback, practitioners may need some background about the OPPE program, including its purpose, who is involved, and the processes and reasoning behind the indicator and threshold selections. Explain these areas in an invitation letter to participate in the pilot group.

Who will participate in the pilot group?

The pilot group should be a small group of no more than 20 practitioners that represent various specialties and departments in the hospital. Here are a few sample pilot group options:

- Medical executive committee (MEC)

- Department/service line chairs

- Practitioner members of the quality or utilization review committee

- Multidisciplinary peer review committee

- Credentials committee

- A few specialties from medicine, surgery, and/or OB/GYN

- A small sample of practitioners from each major specialty

Prior to providing sample reports to the target group, perform a data integrity audit to ensure that the OPPE results conform to the original data collection specifications for each indicator. Leadership has agreed on the original indicator specifications and previously acknowledged defects, imperfections, or other attribution issues that may be inherent in the indicator. Medical staff leaders and the OPPE task force previously vetted and resolved these issues, so they are not the subject of pilot testing. Pilot testing is an attempt to isolate the feedback provided by the target group to evaluate organization, layout, instructions for the evaluator, and other elements intended to assist the target audience in productively using the report.

 © 2011 HCPro, Inc.

If you have a staggered OPPE report delivery process in which a group of practitioners are reviewed at once (based on specialty or another categorization), get several rounds of feedback in a short amount of time if you have the resources to review the feedback quickly and make the appropriate updates before delivering the next set of reports.

Getting feedback on the OPPE program

The OPPE task force should consider how it wants to implement the feedback process. The likelihood is that if the task force does not create a structured and efficient process to guide the feedback, it may not receive feedback at all. Should the request for feedback come from a respected medical staff leader? Should feedback go back to a medical staff leader? Should the task force establish deadlines? What is the best way to create accountability among practitioners? The OPPE task force should consider all of these questions as it creates a feedback loop.

The following are a few options for obtaining feedback:

- Written survey

- Electronic survey

- One-on-one meetings over the phone or in person (this can be time-consuming)

- Scheduled committee or department meeting

- Group discussion (focus group)

Although surveys do not facilitate rich discussion and collaboration, they are the most efficient way to gather feedback, and they provide quantitative and qualitative results that are easy to aggregate.

Sometimes a meaningful review requires a group discussion, and a focus group yields the best results. A focus group format enables the OPPE task force to obtain feedback from a group of users in a single setting. It also ensures that there is an opportunity for feedback on issues that may not have been included on a survey or questionnaire. A focus group composed of medical staff leaders (i.e., the MEC) is a great opportunity to educate leadership about the reports, thus engendering their support.

If the organization already has an OPPE reporting process in place, consider holding off on providing these reports until the new OPPE reports have been finalized. There may be times when the task force must provide two sets of reports for the pilot group to compare, although this is not ideal if practitioners are strapped for time and reviewing multiple reports may not be conducive to their schedules. Feedback received from testing should be forwarded to the OPPE task force for consideration and further improvement to the program or associated tools.

Selecting Tools to Compile Report Data

Arguably one of the biggest challenges with OPPE is that indicator data are stored in multiple systems. Some are extracted from technology systems, and others are manually captured. This poses a problem when attempting to create easy-to-use reports. The OPPE task force must determine a process for compiling indicators from various sources into one manageable report. Technology can facilitate and automate report production. First consider in-house technologies: can any of the existing systems produce reports in the format needed for OPPE?

Purchasing OPPE software can be costly. However, if you decide to evaluate the commercially available options, keep in mind that the software selected needs to be capable of fully supporting the work product, including aggregation and trending of data. Start with the end in mind. What do you want to do and can the vendor meet your needs? Create a specific list of "must haves" and "nice to haves." Use a document such as the one presented in Figure 9.3 to organize identified software requirements. You can also insert the table into a request for proposal to summarize user requirements.

FIGURE 9.3

SAMPLE SOFTWARE VENDOR REQUIREMENT CHART

Item number	Required functionality	Priority	Vendor response

Priority key:

1. Critical function: absolute requirement
2. Improve functionality
3. Future requirement

Vendor response key:

1. Available, currently installed
2. Available, but not installed
3. Under development with projected release date
4. Not available, no plans to develop

Determine your "must haves" by answering the following questions:

- Can the software incorporate data (import or accept exports) from other systems in the organization and blend the multiple indicators generated manually and in IT systems into one source? How efficient are the interface capabilities?

- Does the software allow for easy and efficient edits and additions?

- Does the software allow for effective printing of key components of the OPPE program, such as multiple thresholds and specialty-specific reports?

- Do you want a completely electronic, environmentally friendly OPPE process? Does the software facilitate a paperless process? If physician evaluators will view reports electronically, how complex is this to accomplish and how much training will be required?

- Can the software complete simple calculations and/or create graphs and charts?

As you evaluate software vendors, include stakeholders who will support the OPPE program and use the software on a daily basis in the decision-making process. Rushing the decision-making process or making the decision based only on cost considerations increases the chance that the software will not meet your needs or technical requirements. Consider the functionality of the technology and how well it aligns with your immediate needs. When viewing software demos, consider what you want the OPPE reports, its structure, and components to look like, and use this as your guide to ask the appropriate questions of potential vendors. Also evaluate the vendors' best practice approaches to data aggregation and reporting, as you may learn something valuable that you can incorporate into your program, whether you purchase their software or not.

New software can be a huge investment for an organization, so the OPPE task force and others lobbying for the system should be prepared to demonstrate the return on investment in terms of time saved (including full-time equivalents), improved effectiveness, and other benefits realized as a result of using the new product.

If off-the-shelf technology is not an option, consider a homegrown option that will bring together various data for indicators. This might include spreadsheets or databases. However, an organization may find that it will expend far more resources in developing and supporting a homegrown system than purchasing a software program from a vendor.

In order to index or assign data to each practitioner, you will need a common data field (in other words, one data element that is shared across all systems). This can be the practitioner ID, practitioner name (for aggregated data), the patient account number, or another patient encounter identifier (if you have the nonaggregate, detailed data). The key is to ensure that the data element matches between the various systems (typically, the practitioner ID and patient account numbers are the most reliable).

For example, you may obtain readmission, length of stay, and complications rates from a report writing system exported into a spreadsheet. You may also have board certification, continuing education credits, and peer complaints captured manually in separate spreadsheets. You need a common data field in order to tie all these indicators together to create a single report. If the practitioner ID is in every file, your IT department can import these data into a database and merge them together. You could certainly do this manually in spreadsheets using a formula, but depending on the size of the files, it may take a long time. The following tip box provides a formula for use with a spreadsheet to merge data from various reports.

TIP

Many hospitals use Microsoft® Excel® as their spreadsheet program. If you use Excel, you can use the VLOOKUP formula to merge data from various reports. The following is the Excel formula syntax for VLOOKUP:

VLOOKUP(lookup_value,table_array,col_index_num,range_lookup) Lookup_value:

The value to search in the first column of the table array. *Lookup_value* can be a value or a reference. If *lookup_value* is smaller than the smallest value in the first column of *table_array*, VLOOKUP returns the *#N/A* error value.

Table_array: Two or more columns of data. Use a reference to a range or a range name. The values in the first column of *table_array* are the values searched by *lookup_value*. These values can be text, numbers, or logical values. Uppercase and lowercase text is equivalent.

Col_index_num: The column number in *table_array* from which the matching value must be returned. A *col_index_num* value of 1 returns the value in the first column in *table_array*; a *col_index_num* value of 2 returns the value in the second column in *table_array*; and so on. If the *col_index_num* value is:

- Less than 1, VLOOKUP returns the *#VALUE!* error value.

- Greater than the number of columns in *table_array*, VLOOKUP returns the *#REF!* error value.

Source: http://office.microsoft.com/en-us/excel-help/vlookup-HP005209335.aspx.

© 2011 HCPro, Inc.

Delivering OPPE Reports to Practitioners

Creating a Timeline for Delivering OPPE Reports

The frequency with which a medical staff services department (MSSD) or quality department distributes OPPE reports depends on what body certifies or accredits the organization. For example, organizations accredited by The Joint Commission have less leeway in setting the time frame for reviews because Joint Commission requirements for OPPE are very prescriptive. The Joint Commission has repeatedly stated that 12-month intervals reflect a "periodic" process rather than an "ongoing" process and offers examples of three-, six-, and nine-month cycles on its website.

Alternatively, Det Norske Veritas (DNV) does not prescribe a specific period for performance review. DNV only requires that the hospital review individual practitioner performance data at reappointment or renewal of privileges.

When deciding how often to distribute OPPE results, do not focus on how often the medical staff can produce data, but rather on how much time is needed to complete a cycle of data production and evaluation and distribute the results. For example, producing OPPE reports quarterly may be feasible from a report generation perspective, but that is only one part of the entire evaluation cycle. The organization must build in sufficient time to evaluate and distribute reports. Logistical challenges and organizational resources may heavily influence the frequency of reviews.

Regardless of the frequency your medical staff selects, align the timelines for OPPE and recredentialing. Recredentialing typically happens every two years and OPPE reports contain the data necessary for recredentialing, so having them occur at the same time will reduce duplicated work and save time. For example, many organizations perform an OPPE review every eight months because it dovetails nicely with a 24-month reappointment cycle. Consider the examples of the ineffective and effective timelines in Figures 10.1 and 10.2.

Another option is to stagger the delivery of reports by specialty or groups of practitioners rather that delivering OPPE reports to all practitioners at once. This gives medical staff the opportunity to spread out the work effort and integrate performance improvement initiatives with the OPPE report delivery. The MSSD also can review larger or more challenging specialties during less hectic months. Figure 10.3 is a sample timeline for staggered report distribution by specialty.

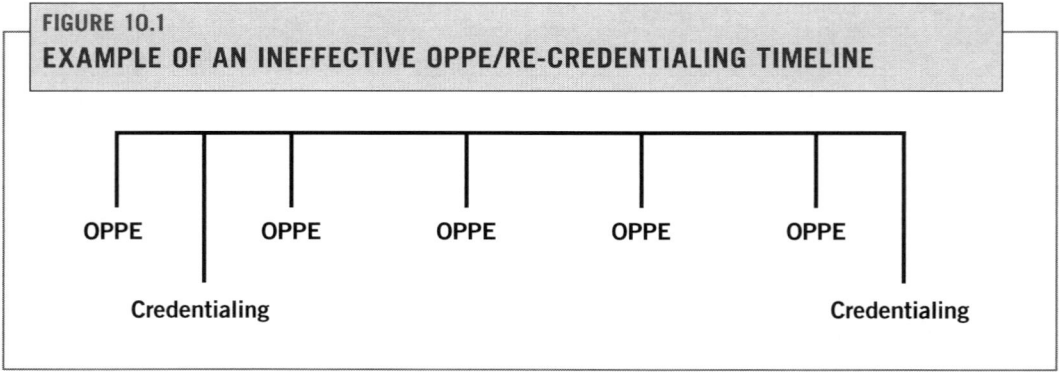

FIGURE 10.1

EXAMPLE OF AN INEFFECTIVE OPPE/RE-CREDENTIALING TIMELINE

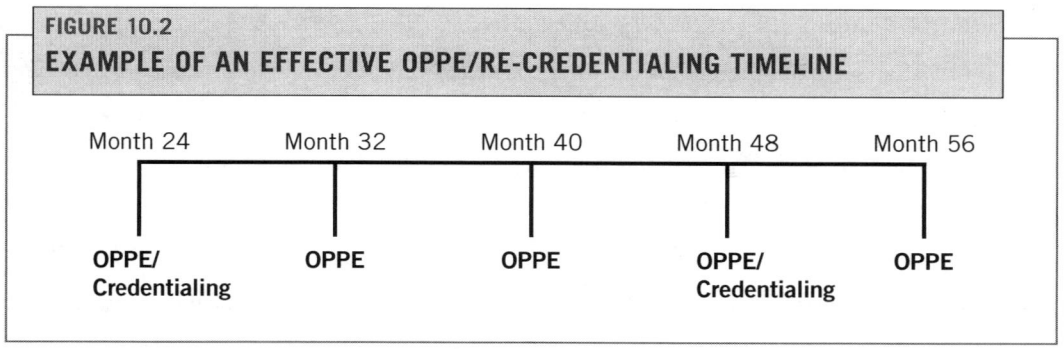

FIGURE 10.2

EXAMPLE OF AN EFFECTIVE OPPE/RE-CREDENTIALING TIMELINE

| Month 24 | Month 32 | Month 40 | Month 48 | Month 56 |
| OPPE/ Credentialing | OPPE | OPPE | OPPE/ Credentialing | OPPE |

FIGURE 10.3

SAMPLE TIMELINE FOR REPORT DISTRIBUTION BY SPECIALTY

Specialty	Cycle 1	Cycle 2	Final review
Anesthesiology	January	June	Medical director, Anesthesiology
Hospitalists	February	July	VPMA/CMO
Diagnostic imaging	March	August	Medical director, Radiology
Podiatry	March	August	Clinical service chair
Nephrology	March	August	Clinical service chair
Urology	March	August	Clinical service chair
Neurology	March	August	Clinical service chair
Family practice	April	September	Clinical service chair of medicine
Internal medicine	April	September	Clinical service chair
Cardiology	May	November	Clinical service chair

Note that the largest groups (Anesthesiology and Hospitalists) are reviewed alone, whereas several smaller specialties are on the March/August cycle.

Staffing support for preparing and distributing reports

Preparing and distributing OPPE reports is usually a collaborative effort between the quality department and the MSSD. However, the tasks each department perform vary depending on the hospital's structure. The quality department may prepare the reports because it has access to a majority of the data, and the MSSD may distribute reports because it has a closer relationship to the practitioners. Alternatively, quality and other departments may send data to the MSSD to collate into reports and deliver to practitioners. Another option is that the quality department or MSSD accesses the software that produces the reports, and prepares and distributes the reports.

Methods of Distributing OPPE Reports

The decision of whether the hospital will routinely distribute OPPE reports to individual privilege holders is not one that should be taken lightly. In large hospitals, distributing reports to all privilege holders may involve thousands of practitioners. If an organization elects to routinely distribute OPPE reports to all practitioners, it will need to carefully consider distribution options, as the approach selected will affect the resources required to fulfill that goal.

The method in which you distribute OPPE reports to practitioners will vary based on the medical staff culture and the resources available. Most hospitals print and distribute reports manually, but there are several other options. Figure 10.4 outlines common strategies for distributing OPPE reports.

Some of the distribution methods described in Figure 10.4 can be resource intensive and may not be feasible, depending on the size of the organization and the resources allocated to the OPPE program. The organization might find it beneficial to limit face-to-face reviews only for practitioners who have potentially adverse OPPE results.

FIGURE 10.4

COMMON METHODS FOR DELIVERING OPPE REPORTS TO PHYSICIANS

Method	Advantages	Disadvantages
Snail mailing reports to practitioners' offices or addresses on record	• Hard copies are easy to review quickly • Tenured physicians are often most accustomed to paper reports • Practitioners are not required to learn a new technology	• Drilling down into case level detail is not immediately available • Because reports are in hard copy, it is difficult to identify root causes of issues • Practitioners' questions result in additional data pulls by an analyst, which is time consuming, provides delayed feedback to the practitioner, and the repetitive work is draining on resources • Requires time to print reports, place them in envelopes, and label them • May be expensive, and there may be concerns regarding confidentiality as mailed performance information may be read by others • Does not facilitate partnership in improvement initiatives

 © 2011 HCPro, Inc.

FIGURE 10.4

COMMON METHODS FOR DELIVERING OPPE REPORTS TO PHYSICIANS (CONT.)

E-mailing reports	• Reduces time and staff effort needed to print and mail reports manually • Ability to track delivery of reports through the use of receipts or notices when practitioners open their e-mails.	• Not all physicians have e-mail addresses or may not routinely check e-mail unless the organization has transitioned the entire medical staff to electronic business correspondence • Many of the same disadvantages of mailing hard copies of reports
Hand-deliver reports to practitioners during medical staff or department meetings	• Encourages collaboration between physicians as it shows them that their peers are receiving the same data • May facilitate discussion on specialty specific metrics for future reports	• Not all physicians attend meetings (although some hospitals have managed to entice physicians in creative ways)
Electronic reporting using Web-based applications or Web portals	• Interactive reports allow for easy drill down and root cause analysis • As new reports are available an automated e-mail could be generated to practitioners inviting them to review their reports at their leisure	• Requires physician-centric technology, which is costly • Learning a new technology is time consuming, and physicians often do not have the luxury of time unless they are already accustomed to conducting credentialing and privileging activities via a Web portal

FIGURE 10.4

COMMON METHODS FOR DELIVERING OPPE REPORTS TO PHYSICIANS (CONT.)

		• If practitioners are not adequately trained to access and interpret electronic reports, they may misinterpret the results • Does not facilitate interactive discussion on improvement
Face-to-face meetings with medical staff leaders or invitations to practitioners to stop by the MSSD or quality department to review their results at their leisure during reappointment processing	• Reduces miscommunication and allows for improved physician relationships • Serves to build relationships and collaborative understanding of organizational initiatives and the practitioners' role in improvement • Helps to gain consensus on OPPE and FPPE policies • Facilitates continual tracking on improvement initiatives pertinent to the practitioner • Allows for engagement and discussion regarding support the practitioners may need to reach desired outcomes • Facilitates the discovery and sharing of best practices among practitioners	• Resource intensive and time-consuming • Requires a skilled clinical practitioner with knowledge of clinical practice and the ability to discuss case-level detail • If one-on-one meetings are mandatory, it would require that the organization identify consequences of nonattendance

© 2011 HCPro, Inc.

TIP

Some organizations have transitioned to electronic communication and no longer send business correspondence to practitioners via mail. At these organizations, using electronic communication may even be a condition of membership and/or privileges, and the medical staff's bylaws or rules and regulations should outline the expectations for electronic communications. Reiterate the expectations for using electronic communication during initial appointment when practitioners must supply an e-mail address on the application form and sign an acknowledgment that the e-mail address will be the principle address used for business correspondence. The expectation to maintain a current e-mail address with the organization can be reinforced at reappointment as well, or the organization may require that all privilege holders use an e-mail address provided by the hospital or health system.

For example, some organizations send practitioners a secure link to a Web portal where practitioners submit electronic applications and privilege form requests. The MSSD can post OPPE data on the same Web portal for practitioners to access. Send practitioners the link to the website along with directions on how to find and access the most recently published OPPE report. The website should include information that would normally be present on a cover letter and a box that practitioners must check off to acknowledge that they received the information.

Regardless of the OPPE report delivery process, it is important to provide practitioners with a phone number or e-mail address where they can direct questions or concerns.

Evaluating Performance and Engaging Practitioners in Performance Improvement Conversations

OPPE reports are the foundation for evaluating practitioner performance and making organizational improvements through targeted conversations with practitioners. The OPPE task force must create a systematic approach for reviewing and evaluating practitioner performance and engaging practitioners in performance improvement (PI) that the medical staff can implement and sustain. Developing a review process and conducting PI conversations with practitioners involves the following steps:

- Creating a process for reviewing OPPE reports

- Identifying common and special cause variation

- Differentiating between organizational process deficiencies and physician performance issues

- Preparing for critical practitioner conversations

- Responding to practitioner questions

- Turning complaints into productive feedback

Staffing the OPPE Review

Before delving into the details of the OPPE report review process, it is important to note that hospitals must adequately staff OPPE reviews in order for them to be successful. OPPE and focused professional practice evaluations (FPPE) have increased the need for additional specialized support for the medical staff services department (MSSD). Every hospital with an OPPE program should have enough people with appropriate qualifications to conduct OPPE reviews and answer questions from practitioners and medical staff leaders responsible for reviewing performance data. One of the worst things that an organization can do to medical staff leaders is hand them a stack of reports of which 95% require no action; it creates busy work and wastes leaders' time and may desensitize them to the importance of OPPE. Medical staff leadership has already provided the OPPE task force guidance for reviewing the results pertaining to a particular threshold. This implies that any reports brought to their attention should be an exception to that threshold. However, check to be sure your hospital's policies and procedures allow implementation of such a process.

The good news is that FPPE and OPPE programs are becoming more meaningful, and as a result, they are having more positive effects on the quality of care. However, this also presents challenges to organizations because traditional approaches to supporting these programs are no longer feasible. More MSSDs find it necessary to modify their approaches to providing staff support to the medical staff organization. MSSDs must ensure support staffs have expertise in clinical quality improvement. Consider the following support staff strategies:

- Partner medical staff services professionals (MSP) with quality improvement or peer review professionals to support competency management programs. This strategy has promise, but because each department has its own reporting structure, the priorities of each group and how each group perceives its role may not always align. To be successful, this approach requires clearly defined procedures and work flow across the two groups. Additionally, the managers of the two collaborating departments must be committed to measuring the results of their mutual efforts to support the competency management program.

- Merge the MSSD and quality improvement department to consolidate management of the two departments to ensure absolute alignment of working relationships, work flow, priorities, and goals.

- Incorporate clinical staff into the MSSD to help evaluate clinical competence and privilege requests. For example, RNs who work in the MSSD bring a clinical eye to the evaluation of credentialing, privileging, OPPE, and FPPE and can help facilitate those reviews along with medical staff leaders.

There is no magic staffing ratio for these types of scenarios. The resources required to support the program are directly related to the scope of the entire competency management program (not just OPPE), the structure of the medical staff organization (divisions vs. departments), and the degree to which the organization can effectively automate tasks.

Creating a Review Process

Establishing a structure for reviewing OPPE reports can be challenging; it is resource-intensive and time-consuming to interpret data. The medical staff drives the OPPE process; however, medical staff leaders often do not have adequate time to review every single report with the necessary level of detail. Effective OPPE review processes involve the administrative departments that support OPPE, such as the MSSD, PI department, or the quality department. This chapter outlines a process considered a best practice, and organizations may modify this process to fit its unique needs.

The sample evaluation process described in the following sections involves three key roles: the administrative evaluator, medical staff leader, and a clinical PI analyst. The administrative evaluator is a clinical or nonclinical staff member who supports the MSSD or quality department and typically performs the initial review of the OPPE reports. The medical staff leader is typically a physician leader, such as a department chair or chief, medical director or chief medical officer (CMO). He or she performs the second review of reports, focusing on practitioners whose OPPE reports indicate that there may be a performance issue. The clinical PI analyst is usually a RN or other individual with a clinical background from the MSSD or PI department dedicated to quality, performance improvement, and OPPE. Clinical PI analysts use their clinical knowledge to review clinical data and support medical staff leaders throughout the OPPE process.

Not all organizations can have an individual fully dedicated to this function, but it is a best practice because it allows for a detailed review of detailed reports with a clinical eye. This individual can also perform the functions of the administrative evaluator if the OPPE process is set up in such a manner.

Phase 1: Administrative department analyst reviews the data

As shown in Figure 11.1, the administrative evaluator (from the MSSD, PI, or quality department), reviews the results of each indicator in the reports and pulls out practitioners whose indicators fall outside the established performance thresholds, as well as practitioners with insufficient data to produce a report. If the administrative evaluator does not have a clinical background, he or she should run questions or concerns by clinical staff, such as the clinical PI analyst, or an RN from the quality department, who is better versed in clinical nomenclature and ascertaining case-level information.

FIGURE 11.1

SAMPLE PHASED APPROACH TO REVIEWING OPPE REPORTS

Administrative evaluator reviews results
(MSSD, quality, or PI departments)

- Separate providers into outliers and nonoutliers by indicator based on established performance thresholds
- Review details on outlier metrics by examining case-level detail when available
- Determine whether outlier status is a result of warranted or unwarranted variation and discover the root causes of issues
- Flag providers with unwarranted variation for further review with medical staff leaders

Medical staff leaders review results
(Department/service line chairs, MEC, CMO)

- Review/approve nonoutlier reports at once
- Review outliers closely with clinical PI analyst
- Identify providers who require FPPE based on established triggers

Deliver reports to practitioners
(all privileged providers/ advanced practice professionals as outlined in bylaws and OPPE policy)

- Practitioners review reports and
- Practitioners are encouraged to contact appropriate medical staff leader or other contact with questions and concerns
- Practitioners referred to the FPPE process meet with medical staff leaders to discuss the FPPE plan

---

When the administrative evaluator identifies an outlier, he or she needs to determine whether the outlier status is a result of a true performance issue or a flaw in the data. The administrative evaluator should review the case-level detail and/or other relevant information to identify the root cause(s) of the performance issue and share it with the appropriate medical staff leaders. If medical staff leaders find that a data problem caused the practitioner to be flagged as an outlier, the appropriate individuals should address the new data integrity issues before sharing reports with other practitioners.

© 2011 HCPro, Inc.

Ensure that the outlier status is valid and justifiable before sharing results with practitioners. Scrutinize the data to prevent practitioners from finding errors in their reports and becoming defensive or angry. After all, this is their livelihood being examined and inaccurate analysis could compromise their long-term relationships and the success of their practices. If the OPPE task force shares an inaccurate report with practitioners, it not only risks alienating the practitioner who received the inaccurate information, but also other practitioners once word gets around that there are data integrity issues in the OPPE process. Once the trust is lost, it is hard to gain back.

Phase 2: Medical staff leaders review the data

In the second tier, a medical staff leader conducts a review of the OPPE reports. To make this review efficient, the administrative evaluator should divide the reports into two or three categories before turning them over to the evaluator. The first category includes all practitioners who are within acceptable thresholds for all indicators or those whose outlier results are tied to data integrity issues (which are addressed and resolved and, if necessary, reported to the OPPE task force). This batch of practitioners typically passes easily through the OPPE process, and the medical staff leaders can sign off on the reports without conducting a detailed review.

Alternatively, some organizations do not have medical staff leaders review reports that fall within acceptable parameters because there are no identified areas of concern. During threshold selection, medical staff leaders and future physician evaluators should provide oversight and direction regarding which reports require their thoughtful consideration and review and which do not. The administrative evaluator can present medical staff leaders with a summary report listing practitioners who had no reported variances.

The second category of reports encompasses practitioners who fall outside the performance thresholds. The reports for these practitioners include additional information and possible explanations for outlier status so that medical staff leaders understand the context. The medical staff leader evaluators decide whether these practitioners necessitate further review or intervention based on the organization's FPPE policy.

The administrative evaluator may further divide the second category into two subcategories: one that encompasses practitioners who require FPPE and another that includes physicians who would benefit from performance improvement efforts but may not require FPPE.

Phase 3: Share reports with practitioners

The Joint Commission does not require that organizations share OPPE reports with practitioners; however, if organizations hold practitioners accountable for their performance, sharing performance data with practitioners is only fair. If organizations don't share performance data with physicians, they don't give practitioners the opportunity to improve.

Many hospitals print individual OPPE reports for medical staff leaders to review and sign and include them in the practitioners' credentials file. Some hospitals use software or an online portal to securely distribute OPPE reports to medical staff leader evaluators. Evaluators review and sign the reports electronically.

Regardless of whether the OPPE report is in hard copy or electronic format, it should include the following elements:

- Summary of results

- Specific results of each indicator

- Details on what each indicator measures

- Definitions of thresholds by indicator

- Who to contact should practitioners have questions

When possible, medical staff leaders should meet face-to-face with practitioners requiring FPPE or coaching to discuss their reports rather than mailing or sharing the reports without context or an opportunity for discussion.

Preparing for Critical Practitioner Conversations Regarding Performance Improvement

OPPE is more than simply a process for identifying outlying performers. OPPE should be rooted in continuous performance improvement for the betterment of healthcare. Healthcare reform, particularly the emergence of financial incentives and accountable care compensation methodologies, increases the need for a robust practitioner performance improvement program. OPPE is an opportunity for individual and groups of practitioners to work together to improve their patient care performance.

Participation in the program is not just in the patient's best interest or the organization's best interest. It is also in the practitioner's best interest. Through the OPPE process, practitioners will identify practice pattern variations that affect certain outcomes, which empowers them to fix the problem. For example, a practitioner's long length of stay may be tied to his or her high consultant usage or resource utilization. This is a great opportunity for a medical staff leader to meet with the practitioner to discuss how his or her length of stay is likely affected by other practice patterns. Another example may be that a practitioner uses a particular antibiotic indiscriminately for most patients. This practice may not always be ideal and may lead to long-term repercussions that affect antibiotic stewardship programs. The practitioner may simply not be aware of such issues. Once again, OPPE can be a great opportunity to coach and educate the practitioner about this practice pattern.

Who should lead these conversations?

Considering the size of the medical staff, medical staff leaders may not have the resources to meet with every single practitioner individually. Set an expectation for a manageable number of practitioners to meet with every month or quarter and create a structured process to identify these practitioners. Aim for the practitioners who offer the biggest bang for your buck. Here are a few options:

- High-volume practitioners or groups

- Practitioners who are particularly open to feedback and coaching

- Outliers with opportunities to improve quality or reduce clinically unnecessary uses

- Practitioners affected by particular initiatives brewing at the organizational level

Consider conducting improvement initiatives during department or division meetings. Share reports and discuss groupwide initiatives. Some organizations share aggregate or blinded individual data with the attendees and/or distribute individual reports to practitioners attending these meetings confidentially in sealed envelopes. These meetings should be led by a medical staff leader, such as the chief medical officer or vice president of medical affairs, department chair, chief of staff, chair of the utilization review committee, or a physician champion with a particular strength or interest. Provide group-level feedback, especially when meeting with group practices such as hospitalists to avoid attribution issues.

Partnering medical staff leaders with clinical PI analysts

When a medical staff leader/reviewer plans to meet with a practitioner whose OPPE data indicates a potential problem, it is crucial that the medical staff leader review the data prior to the meeting in order to understand the root causes for the adverse pattern and to present detailed feedback. It is not sufficient to say, "Dr. Smith, your complication rates are too high" and stop there. Dr. Smith may want to improve complication rates but have no idea how to achieve that goal. Instead, it is much more powerful to say, "Dr. Smith, your complication rates are too high. We have reviewed a sampling of your cases, and the good news is that this doesn't appear to be a clinical issue. It appears that the issue is related to documentation and this is how you might fix it."

Using clinical PI analysts to support OPPE data review

Medical staff leaders may not always have the time or expertise for this level of analysis. If this is the case, the medical staff leader may partner with a clinical PI analyst from the quality/PI departments or MSSD, who can analyze the data prior to meetings and provide the leader with a summary of findings. Some organizations dedicate a nurse or someone with a clinical background who has strong analytical skills to physician performance improvement. The role of this individual is to identify clinically meaningful trends—noting both positive practice patterns and areas for improvement that the leader can share with the practitioner under review. Whether medical staff leaders analyze the data or leverage additional support, their meetings will be more productive if they prepare beforehand.

The clinical PI analyst can be critical to the OPPE process. He or she must have the skills necessary to manage the database or platform used for OPPE. The individual is accountable for working with the health information management/medical record clinical abstractors and/or coders to understand data that interface with or feed the system. If the hospital has an electronic medical record (EMR), the clinical PI analyst may work with individuals responsible for EMRs to automate data collection as a byproduct of care. He or she is also responsible for coordinating all physician PI data and working continuously to ensure the accuracy of that data.

When it is time to bring OPPE reviewers on board, the clinical PI analyst compiles the practitioner profiles or performs the second tier review. He or she may also share the results of the case-level review of metrics with the medical staff leader prior to engaging in a discussion with individual practitioners.

The clinical PI analyst and medical staff leaders may work together to determine a practitioner's opportunities for improvement, next steps, and metrics to be monitored for improvement as the OPPE program continues to evolve. At the end of the first meeting, the clinical PI analyst should establish follow-up dates to revisit OPPE and the particular results. Document the outcomes of these conversations. The documentation may be as simple as, "No variation noted, no modification in privileges recommended."By documenting conversations, the clinical PI analyst can demonstrate the return on investment for both practitioner PI initiatives and the clinical PI analyst.

DOWNLOADABLE RESOURCE AVAILABLE

Download a Sample Performance Conversation Tracking Chart by accessing the link found at the beginning of this book.

 © 2011 HCPro, Inc.

Structuring Conversations With Practitioners

Having collaborative conversations regarding PI is intimidating in any profession and argu-ably more so with healthcare practitioners. Although it is easy to evade such conversations, avoiding them limits the benefits realized from the OPPE program. Preparing for ambigu-ous or negative reactions may help structure conversations. Consider the following tips:

- Provide positive feedback and review areas for improvement

- Understand the practitioner's perspective, which is typically similar to the stages of grief: denial, anger, rationalization, and finally, acceptance

- Foster an environment focused on collaborative curiosity and problem solving rather than presenting a conclusion without discussion by using the SOAP (subject, object, assess, plan) framework

- Be prepared to answer the following question from the practitioner: "So what do you want me to do?"

Each of these strategies is discussed in more detail in the following sections.

Provide positive feedback and areas for improvement

Although including positive feedback and areas for improvement in the conversation might seem obvious, it is easy to get carried away and focus only on the negative aspects of per-formance and forget about what the practitioner does well. It is always best to start with the positive feedback. Share a few key areas where the practitioner performs particularly well, followed by potential improvement opportunities. The more specific the feedback, the more likely the practitioner will remember and respond to it. Focus on the opportunities that are easy wins and offer the highest returns. Keep in mind that organizational inefficiencies or data integrity issues—not the practitioner—may be the causes of some issues. The medical staff leader leading the discussion should take responsibility for non-practitioner–related issues and fix them.

Understand the practitioner's perspective

Understanding and anticipating the practitioner's reaction to performance improvement conversations helps medical staff leaders develop their responses. The following are common reactions and strategies to manage in-the-moment communication to help practitioners move through the gradual process of data acceptance.

If a practitioner is in denial about his or her poor performance, he or she may use phrases such as:

- "I am not interested in reviewing this data."

- "I don't need this to help me care for my patients."

If a practitioner is angry about his or her poor performance, he or she may use phrases such as:

- "This is not my data."

- "One more administrative tool to get us off staff."

- "This does nothing to improve patient care."

Practitioners may try to rationalize their poor performance, and use phrases such as:

- "Ok, I see the results, but my length of stay is necessary for quality of care."

You will know that practitioners recognize and accept their poor performance when they use phrases such as:

- "I appreciate you sharing this with me. I didn't realize my performance was different from that of my peers. What can I do to improve?"

Focus on curiosity and continued data gathering

The SOAP framework, a commonly used care planning tool, is particularly helpful when discussing areas for improvement. Leaders will have a collaborative exchange considering the subject's (practitioner under review) and the object's perspective (medical staff leader), and fairly assess the situation, and plan for solutions to the problem. To have a positive exchange, it is essential for the medical staff leader to actively listen to the practitioner and ask numerous questions to better understand the practitioner's perspective, rather than stating the problem and solution in one breath.

Structure the conversation in the following manner.

Subject's perspective: For this step, the medical staff leader engages the practitioner in a conversation regarding:

- Individual preferences and practice patterns

- The types and demographics of the patients that he or she treats

- The source of patients (e.g., from his or her practice, emergency department, unattended, no-provider call service)

- The practitioner's use of allied health professionals

This conversation will help the medical staff leader gain insight into the practitioner's performance drivers, common referral patterns, and other individuals involved in performance outcomes. During follow-up conversations, the medical staff leader should use an open-ended question such as "How do you feel about your progress to date?" Continue to ask a variety of questions to gain as much understanding as possible to the practitioner's practice. The more a practitioner shares about his or her practice patterns, the more the conversation will move forward in the spirit of collaborative performance improvement.

Object's perspective: At this step, the medical staff leader shares objective information with the practitioner regarding the OPPE report in a nonjudgmental manner. Foster a nonjudgmental atmosphere by using comments such as "Let's review the case to see where the numbers come from", "Let's talk about the use of resources that may contribute to the high cost in the laboratory," "Let me show you what I have seen," or "Let's look at the results together." Refrain from passing judgment by avoiding use of the first person ("I" rather than "you") and by avoiding references to solutions at this point.

Assessment: The goal is to determine the factors affecting the practitioner's performance and come to a mutually shared performance assessment after resolving discrepancies in the report. Medical staff leaders should frame this conversation by asking probing questions, such as "What affects your performance?" or "What barriers exist that hold back your performance?" Also continue to refrain from judgmental statements to encourage a shared assessment.

Planning: At this point, the objective is to plan for improvement. The goal is to create a mutually agreeable plan, determine the metrics that will be used to monitor ongoing improvement, and determine steps to accomplish the goal. Solicit feedback from the practitioner as to what support he or she needs to improve performance. The medical staff leader and practitioner should clearly outline and agree on the practitioner's expectations and responsibilities.

It is important that during these conversations, medical staff leaders use their body language to communicate their engagement and interest in what the practitioner has to say. When leaders respond to practitioner's concerns in an engaged manner, they espouse the value of actively soliciting feedback directed at improving performance.

Respond to practitioner questions and concerns

The success of a medical staff leader's conversation with a practitioner hinges on how successful the medical staff leader is in reviewing and understanding the information in the report and communicating results to the practitioner under review. Anticipate the practitioner's concerns and what he or she might say in defense of his or her performance. The medical staff leader should acknowledge operational issues or process failures, but he or she should keep the focus on how the practitioner can improve performance. If the conversation goes off track, it is critical for the medical staff leader to get back to the topic at hand. Failure to avoid tangential discussions may lead to blaming and confrontation. The medical staff leader must be clear and straightforward so that the practitioner leaves the discussion with a solid improvement plan.

However, this is easier said than done. Not all practitioners are open to feedback and they may try to take some of the pressure off by:

- Offering excuses that may substantiate their behavior or the results

- "Pointing fingers"

- Exercising blame in an effort to avoid ownership or accountability

- Blaming faulty attribution

- Apologizing

- Accepting responsibility without listening to the message or in an attempt to avoid further conversation

- Digressing from the topic under discussion

The leader must communicate to the practitioner that OPPE is not perfect—there will always be ambiguity in data, attribution, normal variation, and system-related issues that are not practitioner-controlled. However, all of the practitioners also participate in the same program and are subject to review. No one is excluded.

Turn complaints into productive feedback

Despite the medical staff leader's efforts to constructively frame feedback, the practitioner may react as though he or she has been attacked and lash out at the medical staff leader personally ("You are always out to get me") or assert that the data is faulty. It is important for medical staff leaders/evaluators and support staff to remain open to any and all feedback from practitioners, regardless of whether it was delivered in a professional manner. An organization cannot expect practitioners to be receptive to performance review if medical staff leaders and other staff supporting the OPPE process are not receptive to the feedback they receive.

Figure 11.2 provides a few typical examples of complaints that practitioners may offer during the course of an evaluation, along with some tips on how to turn the complaints into productive feedback.

FIGURE 11.2

COMMON PRACTITIONER COMPLAINTS REGARDING THE OPPE PROGRAM

Complaint	Translation	Response or next step
"These are not my cases."	There may be a practitioner attribution error.	Perform an audit to confirm whether an attribution error exists. If an error exists, produce a corrected report for review with the practitioner and thank him or her for bringing it to your attention. If an attribution error does not exist, review raw data with practitioner to assist him or her in understanding the source of the data and establish data integrity. Proceed to explore other reasons why his or her results may be different from his or her peers.
"This does not measure my performance. My patients receive excellent care."	The practitioner under review does not recognize the measure as relevant. In addition, he or she may be focused on negative feedback only and does not recognize that there were other indicators on the OPPE report that may indicate areas where the quality of care provided meets or exceeds expectations.	Share feedback with medical staff leadership and the OPPE task force to confirm that the indicator in question is a valid and important measure of performance across the entire specialty. Communicate the outcome to the practitioner under review. Review comparative results from other peers and ask the question, "Why is your data different?" Attempt to isolate the cause of the variation through case review if necessary. Continue to emphasize areas where OPPE indicators indicate a positive result.

  © 2011 HCPro, Inc. THE COMPLETE GUIDE TO OPPE

FIGURE 11.2

COMMON PRACTITIONER COMPLAINTS REGARDING THE OPPE PROGRAM (CONT.)

Complaint	Translation	Response or next step
"Your report does not account for the fact that my patients are sicker than other practitioners' patients."	The practitioner under review is asserting that the report did not adequately capture the complexity or acuity of his or her patients.	Is the indicator severity adjusted? If it is then it does take into account that patients are sicker. Otherwise, compare the CMI to peers and review the indicator definition with the practitioner. Ask him or her for thoughts on how the specificity of the indicator can be improved to better account for patient acuity. Communicate any feedback received to medical staff leaders and the OPPE task force. Emphasize that the tool is a screening tool meant to ask the question, "Why are your scores different from your peers?" His or her response may assist the evaluator in understanding the practitioner's scores. If the practitioner or evaluator requests, the organization can drill down and confirm why the results reported for this practitioner are different than his or her peers.
"This does not apply to me or my practice. My practice is different from everyone else's."	The practitioner believes that he or she should be exempted from a particular performance measure.	Review specific reasons why the practitioner feels that the indicator is not applicable to his or her practice. Solicit a rationale regarding why his or her patients would be subject to a different standard of care or a different expected outcome to assess the validity of the claim. Communicate results to evaluators for further discussion.

 © 2011 HCPro, Inc.

FIGURE 11.2

COMMON PRACTITIONER COMPLAINTS REGARDING THE OPPE PROGRAM (CONT.)

Complaint	Translation	Response or next step
"The report is full of inaccuracies."	The practitioner has identified some specific defect in the data provided.	Solicit the <u>specific</u> defect. 1. If the defect is unexpected or not previously identified, evaluate and resolve any data integrity issues. 2. If the defect was identified as a risk when the indicator was originally selected and the OPPE task force deemed it to be a common/expected factor that would not impede the effective use of the indicator, inform the practitioner. Offer to forward his or her concern to leadership. 3. If the defect is a constant factor across all practitioners to which the indicator is applied, a peer group comparison may help the practitioner under review to understand that he or she is not being singled out and to identify why he or she is different from his or her peers.

 © 2011 HCPro, Inc. THE COMPLETE GUIDE TO OPPE

CHAPTER 12

When OPPE Leads to FPPE

The focus of this book is OPPE. However, because OPPE can lead to or trigger focused professional practice evaluation (FPPE), it is both relevant and beneficial to provide at least a brief overview of FPPE. FPPE is a process whereby an organization takes a closer look at a practitioner's clinical practice to assess his or her clinical competence. FPPE can be performed in response to three circumstances. First, it occurs when the medical staff initially grants a physician privileges. Second, it may be triggered when the medical staff has a question or concern about a practitioner's clinical competence, which might arise during OPPE or at any other time. Third, FPPE may be an option used for evaluating the competency of low-volume practitioners. Performaing a case review oftentimes is the best option for pracititoners who have only a few patients at the hospital.

FPPE for Initial Privileges

FPPE is a process whereby an organization evaluates and confirms the privilege-specific competence of a practitioner who does not have documented evidence of competently performing the requested privilege at the hospital. FPPE replaced a predecessor concept called "focused review." Previously, the medical staff only conducted a focused review when it had doubts or concerns about a privileged practitioner's clinical competence and ability to provide safe, high quality patient care. Currently, The Joint Commission requires hospitals to perform FPPE whenever they grant new privileges to practitioners. Organizations must conduct a period of FPPE and confirm clinical competence of all initially requested privileges. It might be helpful to think of FPPE as a replacement of the more general performance assessment previously completed during the provisional period review, except that FPPE is targeted at specific areas of privileging and is more diagnostic in nature than a general provisional review. Organizations can no longer assume clinical competence based on the process of credentialing and privileging verification and the contents of the credentials file. They have to prove it!

FPPE for Clinical Practice Concerns

The second situation that triggers the FPPE process involves the identification of potential practice concerns, behaviors, or an inability to perform a procedure identified during OPPE or at any other time. The rationale for performing OPPE is similar to the rationale for performing FPPE. Organizations used to simply assume that "no news is good news." If the medical staff leaders did not hear anything bad about a practitioner, then that must mean that the practitioner provided acceptable quality care. OPPE changed this approach. Hospitals are no longer permitted to assume that because a practitioner's quality improvement file is "empty," he or she must be okay. They have to prove it, not just once, but on an ongoing basis. The Joint Commission now expects hospitals to have data that affirms or proves ongoing clinical competence of currently privileged practitioners.

The results of OPPE may raise concerns about a physician's current clinical competence, practice behavior, ability to perform a procedure, or the quality of care provided by a particular practitioner. If a practitioner's performance falls below a particular threshold on an OPPE report, or an incident raises concerns about clinical competence, the medical staff should perform FPPE to find the root cause.

When an OPPE report notes potentially adverse information, the medical staff leader (such as a department chair) has several follow-up options available. For example, a department chair may decide that the practitioner requires further education and simply sends the practitioner a letter to remind him or her of a particular practice expectation or policy or recommend specific continuing medical education related to the procedure or topic in question.

However, there are other situations in which the medical staff leader evaluator may consider recommending FPPE, such as the following:

- An evaluator has questions about whether an anecdotal incident is common to a practitioner's day-to-day practice or an isolated event.

- An evaluator may want to confirm whether there are legitimate reasons why a particular practitioner's indicator value is different from the peer group. For example, a practitioner's results may have adverse selection that was not mitigated during risk adjustment. This could include a higher average age of patients than peers or more patients presenting with comorbid conditions like diabetes.

- An evaluator may request FPPE to take a closer look at practice patterns and confirm whether a larger performance problem that requires an intervention exists.

- The practitioner may have insufficient clinical activity to produce a data-driven report, so the evaluator may request FPPE in an effort to obtain an assessment of the few cases available for review.

- The medical staff must determine whether current medical staff members who have requested additional privileges or privileges to perform new procedures are competent to perform them independently.

- The medical staff must evaluate the competence of a practitioner who has re-entered medicine after an extended leave of absence or has been practicing in a setting that does not have the level of acuity of hospital-based care.

- The medical staff must assess the performance of low- or no-volume practitioners.

- Organizations may find it helpful to incorporate the potential triggers for FPPE into their OPPE reports. OPPE reports can be designed not only to provide information to evaluators but also to offer a springboard to the next step in the process. Organizations may design their OPPE reports to embed the potential for FPPE into both the report and the recommendation form, which may assist in guiding medical staff leaders toward likely next steps when a physician's performance throws up a red flag. The report itself can also provide a record of the outcome of the review.